The Vaccine Court

The Vaccine Court

The Dark Truth of America's Vaccine Injury
Compensation Program

Wayne Rohde

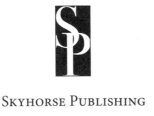

SKYHORSE PUBLISHING

Skyhorse Publishing books may be purchased in bulk at special discounts for sales promotion, corporate gifts, fund-raising, or educational purposes. Special editions can also be created to specifications. For details, contact the Special Sales Department, Skyhorse Publishing, 307 West 36th Street, 11th Floor, New York, NY 10018 or info@skyhorsepublishing.com.

Skyhorse® and Skyhorse Publishing® are registered trademarks of Skyhorse Publishing, Inc.®, a Delaware corporation.

Visit our website at www.skyhorsepublishing.com.

10 9 8 7 6 5 4 3 2 1

Library of Congress Cataloging-in-Publication Data is available on file.

Cover design by Qualcom Design
Cover photo: Thinkstock

Print ISBN: 978-1-62914-452-8
Ebook ISBN: 978-1-63220-169-0

Printed in the United States of America

There has been a betrayal of the promise that was made to parents about how the compensation program would be implemented.
—Barbara Loe Fisher

Contents

Introduction

This book is about the National Vaccine Injury Compensation Program—the vaccine court—from the perspective of families who have experienced firsthand vaccine-related injuries and death and who have filed petitions with the program. The National Childhood Vaccine Injury Act of 1986 (NCVIA) established a no-fault compensation system for vaccine-related injuries or death linked to childhood vaccinations. Several years later, the program would be extended to include vaccinations received by adults. Under this no-fault system, a $0.75 excise tax on each antigen component of a vaccine covered by the program goes into a trust fund account known as the Vaccine Injury Trust Fund.

In this book, I will attempt to highlight and convey the stories of several families who have filed petitions with the NVICP, some of whom won compensation and many of whom have had their cases dismissed. I will discuss some meaningful developments of the NVICP, how the vaccine court handles petitions, the special masters who make decisions on the petitions, and Department of Justice (DOJ) attorneys who defend the government position (the Respondent). I will attempt to present legal decisions in plain English, and I will show how those decisions affect both adults and the parents of vaccine-injured children who have to deal with the process of filing petitions, handle the ongoing process of worrying about the fate of their petition, all amid the constant daily routines of providing care for their children and family members.

The Vaccine Injury Trust Fund provides compensation for victims of vaccine-related injuries and death plus attorney fees and medical expert fees. The ability to sue a vaccine manufacturer directly is not permitted in the United States. Petitioners submit claims of injury or death to the NVICP. When the NVICP was first established, injured parties were required to file petitions with the program and then, if not satisfied with the outcome, they could exit the program and file civil tort-related suits in state or federal court. However, since 2011, the US Supreme Court, ruling in *Bruesewicz v. Wyeth Labs*, eliminated the option, as established by Congress, to exit the program and file suit against the vaccine manufacturer.

Prior to the establishment of the NVICP, parents of children who suffered vaccine-related injuries or death would seek remedy or compensation by filing suit in state or federal court lawsuits. As more vaccines were introduced in the 1970s and 1980s, an increase in vaccine-related injuries and death led to a corresponding increase in vaccine-related tort filings which, due to the cost of litigation, led to a greater threat to the nation's vaccine supply. The diptheria-pertussis-tetanus (DTP) vaccine illustrates the problem manufacturers were having, resulting in their leaving the market, due to presumed high litigation costs and lack of liability insurance, or at least threatening to do so.

Congress passed the NCVIA of 1986 to address the problems that lawsuits presented for both the vaccine manufacturers and, more importantly, the families of injured children. Congress established the program as no-fault compensation to allow petitioners to file claims without having to prove fault on part of the manufacturer. Their petitions are adjudicated in the federal court system known as the Court of Federal Claims.

Also included in the NCVIA was the establishment of the Vaccine Adverse Event Reporting System (VAERS). Congress mandated that health professionals and vaccine manufacturers report specific adverse events that occur after the administration of the vaccine. In 1993, then FDA Commissioner David Kessler, MD, published a report in the *Journal of the American Medical Association* that stated physicians failed to report up to 99 percent of all serious adverse reactions to vaccines and medications.

Under the NCVIA, successful petitioners are entitled to compensation for 1) pain and suffering and emotional distance distress not to exceed $250,000; 2) loss of earnings; 3) non-reimbursable medical expenses and; 4) in the case of vaccine-related death, an award up to a cap of $250,000. Petitioners may file either an on-table or off-table claim for vaccine-related injury. On-table claim refers to petitions in which the child receives a program-covered vaccine and experiences an injury listed in the vaccine injury table within the associated time. An off-table claim, by contrast, is filed in response to an injury, disease, or medical condition that is not listed in the table in relation to the received vaccine. Petitioners who file off-table claims bear the burden of proving by a preponderance of evidence that the vaccine was the cause of the injury or symptoms.

In areas of medical uncertainty, where it is equally probable that the vaccine or another factor caused the injury, the presumption should be for the petitioner and compensate the child's injuries. Most descriptions of the program start with a no-fault compensation program. But in the reality of today's setting, the NVICP is not a no-fault system, but an adversarial, highly litigious court process that Congress intended to stay away from.

Once a petition has been filed, the office of the Division of Vaccine Injury Compensation (DVIC), an agency within the Health Resources and Services Administration, will review and file a Rule 4 report with the court outlining the respondent's legal position and medical interpretation of the filed petition. DOJ attorneys representing the respondent may offer a settlement to be negotiated with the petitioner, concede the injury or death and offer damages, or recommend the court to dismiss the petition. A special master will oftentimes review the Rule 4 report and the petition, conduct teleconference calls with attorneys representing both the petitioner and the respondent, review medical literature, and conduct hearings with medical experts from both sides, all to reach a logical conclusion and publish a decision for compensation or dismiss the petition.

The current standard for proving causation in cases involving off-table injuries comes from the landmark case that was decided in 2005, *Althen v. HHS*. This decision finally provided petitioners more equitable means to prove causation. Prior to *Althen*, the court was inconsistent in its decisions, starting with nearly a blank slate from Congress on how to determine and adjudicate off-table injuries. Some of the early cases were very punitive toward petitioners and created an undue burden regarding causation. Under the *Althen* standard, petitioners must demonstrate causation by providing 1) a medical theory causally connecting the vaccination and the injury; 2) a logical sequence of cause and effect showing the vaccination was the reason for the injury; and 3) an approximate temporal relationship between the vaccination and the injury.

A petitioner who demonstrates all three prongs, or standards, of the *Althen* test is entitled to recover damages unless the respondent shows, also by a preponderance of evidence, that the injury was, in fact, caused by factors unrelated to the vaccine.

Protecting your identity and that of your family's is a high priority for most Americans. In the NVICP, this has become one of the most contentious issues. The Vaccine Act allows a special master, or a judge, to redact certain information from any decision, opinion, or order. Yet even the most generous decision in favor of the petitioner has not gone far enough to protect personal information from being invaded by those individuals and organizations that use this information to intimidate petitioners and discourage the filing of petitions with the NVICP.

As of March 2014, there have been over 15,100 petitions filed with the NVICP; only 3,500 petitions have been awarded compensation; nearly $2.8 billion has been paid to petitioners and their attorneys, and the balance of the Vaccine Injury Trust Fund is somewhere north of $3.4 billion and growing each year.

Chapter 1

How Did We Get Here?

In order for us to properly examine today's National Vaccine Injury Compensation Program, whether to advocate for stronger reform measures or to keep the status quo, or to push for a complete repeal of the existing program, we need to have a better understanding of how and why the NVICP came into existence.

From the middle of the nineteenth century through the early twentieth century, the vaccination policy in the United States was centered around the eradication of smallpox. Out of the struggle against smallpox came the landmark United States Supreme Court ruling in 1905 of *Jacobson v. Massachusetts*.[1]

The facts of the case boil down to a conflict between a single man, Jacobson, and the State of Massachusetts, over whether or not Massachusetts could force Jacobson to be vaccinated. Massachusetts had passed a statute in 1902 requiring all citizens who had not been vaccinated at some point during the past five years to become vaccinated or pay a fine. Jacobson, however, refused both to be vaccinated and to pay the fine. He sued on the argument that the Massachusetts statute infringed on his liberty and sought to have his position supported through Massachusetts law. The Massachusetts Supreme Court ruled against him, however, so he appealed to the United States Supreme Court. They decided against Jacobson, ruling that Jacobson's refusal to accept the vaccination was not so much an act of individual choice as it was an act endangering those around him; He was accepting the benefits of everyone else having received the vaccine without having gotten it himself. Furthermore, this was a situation in which the State had the power to force citizens to act in certain ways in order to protect the common good. The case established the concept of manifold restraints to action which each citizen inherently accepts in being a citizen in order to make the overall society function. There was some dissent, as the decision was a 7–2 decision, but it was accepted, in general, primarily because it was so clearly in favor of the public.[2]

Further, Mr. Jacobson argued that children were exempted by physicians who determined the vaccination was medically contra-indicated; there was no exemption for adults. Mr. Jacobson also wanted to present medical evidence that he had experienced an adverse reaction to a prior vaccination along with medical research undermining the efficacy and safety of vaccination. The high court rejected the offer from Mr. Jacobson.

That ruling upheld the state's right to enforce compulsory vaccination laws. At the time of the ruling, there were eleven states that had mandatory vaccination laws, most to combat the smallpox outbreaks. The ruling also created the first medical exemption under Massachusetts law.

As more vaccines were developed to prevent childhood diseases in the first half of the twentieth century, so, too, did the discussion of how to deal with those who died or were injured from these vaccines.

Despite the tremendous health benefits of vaccinations, according to our medical community, a small percentage of children and adults suffered a variety of injuries as a result of them, ranging from minor fever to anaphylactic shock to death.

In 1955 many people were paralyzed and several died after contracting polio from the Salk polio vaccine. It turned out that 120,000 doses made by Cutter Laboratories in Berkeley contained the live polio virus.[3] In the end, at least 160 children were permanently paralyzed, ten died, and perhaps 40,000 experienced less serious bouts with the virus.[4] The first cases of polio in children who received the tainted vaccine were reported to regulators on April 25, 1955—two weeks after the nation began a drive to vaccinate millions of schoolchildren.[5]

Certain production lots were not made inactive, despite the manufacturers' adherence to federal government standards. This event would come to be named after one of the manufacturers involved in this tragic episode—the Cutter Incident. Many books and legal papers have been written debating the merits of the incident and subsequent legal proceedings. Many of the injured people and their families filed lawsuits against the manufacturers and settled out of court. However, one case did proceed in the courts. *Gottsdanker v. Cutter Laboratories,* on appeal to the California State Supreme Court, upheld a lower court ruling that the manufacturer was not negligent in its design or manufacture of the vaccine because it followed the standards set by our federal government.[6] However, the company was held liable for financial damages because of the harm the vaccine caused.[7]

Because of the general acceptance of the idea that the benefits of vaccination far outweighed these risks, every state adopted measures that required children to receive certain vaccinations prior to entering school. However, as more mandates were placed upon our nation to vaccinate against certain diseases, it became evident that families of injured children needed a legal option to seek compensation for their injuries. Originally, persons who claimed injury as a result of receiving a vaccine relied solely on the civil law tort system for a remedy. The system over time proved to be unsatisfactory for both the vaccine manufacturers and the plaintiffs—those who filed seeking compensation for their injuries. The plaintiff often found the system to be very time-consuming, extremely expensive, and therefore limited to those who would have access to file suit. It was also difficult to determine the exact nature of causation. Vaccine manufacturers also began to feel the impact of the court's ruling in the 1960s and 1970s from *Davis v. Wyeth Labs.*[8]

In *Davis v. Wyeth Labs,*[9] the plaintiff contracted polio after being vaccinated for that disease as part of a nationally sponsored immunization program and sued the manufacturer of the vaccine for, among other things, failure to provide an adequate warning. The jury returned a verdict for the defendant, but the Court of Appeals reversed on the ground that "the manufacturer [had] a duty to warn the consumer (or make adequate provision for his being warned) as to the risks involved."[10]

The Court of Appeals asserted in their ruling in *Davis*:

Here, however, although the drug was denominated a prescription drug it was not dispensed as such. It was dispensed to all comers at mass clinics without an individualized balancing by a physician of the risks involved. In such cases . . . warning by the manufacturer to its immediate purchaser will not suffice. The decision (that on balance and in the public interest the personal risk to the individual was worth taking) may well have been that of the medical society and not that of [the manufacturer]. But just as the responsibility for choice is not one that the manufacturer can assume for all comers, neither is it one that he can allow his immediate purchaser to assume. In such cases, then, it is the responsibility of the manufacturer to see that warnings reach the consumer, either by giving warning itself or obligating the purchaser to give warning.[11]

In 1974, the United States Court of Appeals for the Fifth Circuit, in *Reyes v. Wyeth Labs*,[12] held polio vaccine manufacturers strictly liable for failing to provide product warnings directly to the vaccinees.[13]

The plaintiff in that case contracted polio slightly more than two weeks after she was vaccinated for that disease at a county health clinic. The vaccine was administered by a registered nurse; no physician was present. The nurse who administered the vaccine said that she read the package circular accompanying the vaccine, but did not warn the plaintiff of the risks of vaccination.

The plaintiff sued the manufacturer of the vaccine for, among other things, failure to warn. The defendant argued that it met its duty to warn by inserting an adequate warning—the package circular—in the vials of vaccine, and that *Davis v. Wyeth Labs* was distinguishable because (1) whereas the plaintiff in Davis was vaccinated as part of a mass immunization program, the plaintiff in Reyes was vaccinated at her parents' request; (2) whereas the plaintiff in Davis was vaccinated by a pharmacist, the plaintiff in Reyes was vaccinated by a "public health nurse"; (3) compared to the defendant in Davis, it "played a relatively passive role" in the national immunization program; and (4) unlike the defendant in Davis, it "had no knowledge that the vaccine would not be administered as a prescription drug." 498 F.2d at 1277.

The Reyes court found the defendant's arguments unpersuasive. Embracing the rationale of Davis, the court first observed that "[w]here there is no physician to make an 'individualized balancing . . . of the risks,' . . . the very justification for the [learned intermediary rule] evaporates." The court then rejected the defendant's attempt to distinguish Davis on the facts presented.[14]

The Swine Flu Fiasco of 1976

In January 1976, a soldier died and four other soldiers became ill from influenza at Fort Dix, New Jersey. Health officials were concerned and thought the death and illnesses were caused by a strain of influenza similar to the flu pandemic of 1918, the Spanish Flu, which killed 500,000 American citizens and millions of people around the world.[15] Because of this concern, the public health officials successfully lobbied and encouraged the federal government to start a mass immunization program against influenza.[16] Congress started the mass inoculation program in April 1976 by purchasing over 200 million batches of flu vaccine from manufacturers. It was later determined that the flu strain at Fort Dix was not the Spanish Flu. Neither a swine flu epidemic nor a pandemic materialized.

The tension surrounding the potential liability of vaccine injury was now front and center as insurance companies stopped providing liability insurance to vaccine manufacturers by June 30, 1976.[17] The domino effect continued as vaccine manufacturers balked at providing the needed influenza vaccine without some form of liability protection from our federal government. Could the hoax or hysteria of a flu epidemic have really been caused by an overreaction or 'end-of-the-world-scenario mentality by the insurance companies that provided liability insurance to vaccine manufacturers? What is truly remarkable is the fact that the fear promoted by the insurance industry was never investigated during the debate in Congress. Was the "fear" actually real, or were the insurance companies again using their "frivolous" lawsuits threat, or was it a coordinated effort by the vaccine manufacturers to orchestrate a "perceived" medical threat to get some favorable business-oriented legislation?

In August 1976, Congress passed the National Swine Flu Immunization program, or "Swine Flu Act." This act transferred liability from the vaccine manufacturers and those who administered the vaccine to the federal government for any injuries that resulted from the swine flu vaccine. However, the act still required the federal court system to resolve injury cases. Plaintiffs asserted claims directly against the United States through the Federal Tort Claims Act rather than against the alleged "wrongdoer,"[18] and the United States assumed the liability of manufacturers, distributors, and vaccinators, "Based on any theory of liability . . . including negligence, strict liability in tort, and breach of warranty."[19] The cost of the program to the taxpayers would be $135 million, but it would be advertised to the public as a free vaccine for everyone. As with so many programs in Washington, DC, there is always a hidden cost.

Claimants had an exclusive route to compensation from the federal government for personal injury or death arising from the swine flu vaccine.[20] The bill, introduced by Senator Ted Kennedy, was passed the same day by both houses without meaningful consideration by any committee in either house. During the time the bill passed the House, most congressmen did not even have a copy of it. See 122 Cong.Rec. 26,625-40, 26,793-817 (1976). President Gerald Ford and Congress believed that the legislation had to be passed quickly so that the Swine Flu Program could be implemented in time to protect the population during the winter of 1976–1977.[21]

The federal government quickly halted the immunization program at the end of 1976 after 45 million people were vaccinated and it became clear that the flu pandemic seemed unlikely to develop, and because of side effects to that flu vaccine that became more prominent, such as Guillain-Barré Syndrome and transverse myelitis.[22] Four hundred and fifty people developed the rare Guillain-Barré Syndrome.[23] Thirty people died as a result of the flu vaccination.

The threat never materialized.[24] The panic in 1976 was partly because of the belief—now known to be erroneous—that the 1918–1919 flu pandemic, which killed half a million Americans and as many as fifty million worldwide, was caused by a virus with swine components.[25] Recent research suggests instead that it was avian flu, but that seems unlikely to assuage the current anxiety.[26]

By 1985, the federal government had reportedly paid out over $90 million to settle the many lawsuits as a result of the swine flu inoculation program.[27] However, CBS News, through their *60 Minutes* program, uncovered many disturbing issues about the actions of the federal government and a possible cover-up of policy decisions that turned out to be monumental mistakes. In the *60 Minutes* story, Mike Wallace reported that the federal government paid out a total of $3.5 billion, not the $90 million figure reported by our government and used in several media stories.[28] This discrepancy can be explained as the total amount of compensation that was filed by the claims versus what was actually paid out to settle all claims. The true figure has yet to verified.

Highlighted in the *60 Minutes* program, which aired in November 1979, is the story of Judi Roberts, an assistant principal at a local public school in Lakeland, Florida. She, like forty-five million other Americans, received the flu vaccine. She received her vaccination in November 1976. Within two weeks, she suffered partial paralysis, and one week later, was totally paralyzed. In order to breathe properly, her doctors performed a tracheotomy. Judi's condition improved somewhat, allowing her to be confined to a wheelchair for the first year of her ordeal. She would later regain the ability to walk, with the help of braces for each leg. Her doctors ultimately diagnosed her with Guillain-Barré Syndrome (GBS).

As she began the slow process of recovering from GBS, Judi also began what would be the even slower process of adjudicating her claim in federal court. Judi and her husband, Gene Roberts, filed a claim, seeking $12 million in damages. After researching what actually happened with the soldiers at Fort Dix, she mentioned in the *60 Minutes* report that, had she known what occurred at Fort Dix, she might not have received the flu vaccination.

In the CBS program, viewers were enlightened about the story of Private Lewis. In January of 1976, many of the new recruits at Fort Dix were complaining of symptoms of respiratory illness, much like a common cold. The Army doctor sent throat cultures to the New Jersey Health Lab to determine what type of bug was going around. Meanwhile, Private Lewis left his sick bed to go on a march with his unit. He would later collapse during the march. His sergeant revived Private Lewis with mouth-to-mouth resuscitation. The sergeant would not show any signs of illness; Private Lewis would die a couple of days later.

We need to examine what actually happened, how our government promoted an immunization program, and the consequences of the swine flu fiasco of 1976. The health lab determined the throat cultures of many of the soldiers were the common flu or the common cold. However, the cultures of five soldiers, including Private Lewis, were different. The lab could not determine what type of virus it was, so they sent those cultures to the Centers for Disease Control and Prevention (CDC). Within a few days, the results were sent to Fort Dix. The five soldiers had swine flu. Four of the soldiers, excluding Private Lewis, recovered within a couple of days without a flu vaccination.

The message that was promoted to many Americans was that this strain of flu had the potential to kill millions of people. Judi Roberts understood this to mean, in her words, "If a healthy, active soldier will die from this, then a middle-aged school teacher does not have a prayer."[29] She continued by stating that if she "knew the boy was sick, got up, and participated in a forced march, later collapsed and died, I would have never received the flu shot."[30]

The CDC developed an immunization program led by Dr. David Sencer, the head of the CDC. In the *60 Minutes* report, he stated the following: "The rationale for our recommendation was not on the basis of the death of a single individual, but was on the basis of when we see a change in the characteristics of the influenza virus, it is a massive public health problem for this country."[31]

Remember, the CDC reviewed the five throat cultures and read the report from the New Jersey health lab about the rest of the throat cultures all having the seasonal flu virus commonly seen in the United States. The CDC began the largest mass immunization program based upon the lab results of five cultures that revealed swine flu, not the Spanish flu that killed 500,000 people in this country in 1918–1919.

The immunization program would start October 1, 1976. Between then and December 16, 1976, over 40 million US citizens were vaccinated. Additionally, Department of Defense and Veterans Administration programs accounted for several million more.[32] Immunization rates varied between states and even between cities within states. Houston, Texas, inoculated 10 percent of the adult population while San Antonio immunized one-third of its population. Minnesota led the nation for large states and immunized two-thirds of its adult population, and the first case of GBS was diagnosed there in the third week of November 1976.[33]

Within another week, the state of Minnesota reported to the CDC several more cases of GBS and a couple of fatalities. Other states started to report several cases to the CDC. With these reports, Dr. Sencer, the head of the CDC, consulted with leading influenza experts and neurological experts and concluded that the statistical association of GBS with the influenza vaccine was inconclusive. But they did agree that until the risk was established, it could not be put into a consent form.[34] Dr. Sencer consulted with Dr. Salk, who was in Paris, and all agreed to approach President Ford to stop the immunization program. On December 16, 1976, nearly nine months after the initial announcement of the swine flu immunization program, President Ford agreed to immediately suspend the vaccinations.

Dr. Theodore Cooper, Assistant Secretary for Health in the Department of Health, Education, and Welfare, released a press release later the same day, suspending the immunization program "in the interest of safety of the public, in the interest of credibility, and in the interest of the practice of good medicine."[35] According to Dr. Sencer, there were several reported cases of swine flu around the world, but nothing was confirmed. The most damning question asked by Mike Wallace to Dr. Sencer was the following: "Have you uncovered any other confirmed swine flu cases other than those from Fort Dix?" Dr. Sencer's answer was "No." Was the United States and its 218 million citizens just hoodwinked into believing an epidemic was emerging, when in fact there was no evidence to support the CDC's assertions?

When the immunization program was rolled out, the CDC created a consent form so that every person could have all the information regarding the safety of the swine flu vaccine. What the public did not know was that the flu vaccine described in the consent form was not the same strain as the influenza vaccine that was part of the immunization program. The flu strain vaccine given to most of the people was called X53A.[36] Dr. Sencer, in his interview with Mike Wallace, stated that he did not know if the X53A flu vaccine was ever tested.[37] The consent form that was handed out to those who received the flu vaccine did not mention the adverse reactions or risks involved, such as heart attacks or GBS, but rather mentioned sore arm or a headache.

Dr. Michael Hartwick, leading the surveillance team at the CDC for the swine flu immunization program, reported that there were possibilities of neurological injuries with the swine flu vaccine. Dr. Sencer mentioned that he did not hear of any report of neurological injuries, a claim Dr. Hartwick has called "ridiculous." As hundreds of claims were filed across the country seeking compensation for the injuries from the vaccination, the court system and the Department of Justice brought the entire process to a halt.

In the spring of 1978, the Secretary of Health, Education, and Welfare, Joseph Califano, Jr., promised to cut the bureaucratic red tape for victims suffering from GBS and to pay them quickly. On February 28, 1978, the Judicial Panel on Multidistrict Litigation ordered that all swine flu cases be transferred to the District of Columbia for coordinated and consolidated pretrial proceedings.[38]

Secretary Califano stated the following during the *60 Minutes* interview: "We shouldn't hold them to an impossible or too difficult standard to prove that they were hurt. Even if we pay a few people a couple of thousand dollars that might not deserve it, I think justice requires we promptly pay those people who do deserve it." When asked who was making the decision to be so hardnosed about the claims that had been filed, he continued, "I assume that the Justice Department has been." Today, you could place Secretary Califano's words into the discussion of what is happening in the NVICP.

Anyone who has recently filed a petition in the NVICP will tell you that the attorneys from Justice (DOJ) are hardnosed and extremely difficult to deal with. And with comparisons to the swine flu fiasco nearly thirty-five years earlier, it appears that the DOJ views petitions or claims made by US citizens as a nuisance or inconvenience.

Judi Roberts, in the same *60 Minutes* program, concluded by saying that "if it drags out long enough, people will just give up." Her statement rings just as true today as it did thirty-five years ago. Gene Roberts, Judi's husband, said the following, "I am mad, that my government, because they knew the facts, they did not release those facts, because if they had released them, the people would not have taken the vaccine. And they can come out tomorrow and tell me there is going to be an epidemic, they can drop like flies, because I will not take another shot my government tells me to take."[39]

This created a national movement of not trusting our government, the CDC, and other agencies when it comes to medical issues. The swine flu fiasco came on the heels of a nation still trying to deal with the Watergate scandal. President Carter would later fire Dr. Sencer. And a little-known federal prosecutor named Laura Millman, who would defend the government against many of the swine flu lawsuits, would later be appointed a Special Master in the NVICP.

The federal government and the CDC missed out on one of the great opportunities to study the medical outcomes of all those who were vaccinated with the "swine flu" vaccine, or rather the X53A influenza vaccine. The conclusion to Judi Roberts's story is that she never fully recovered from GBS. She lived the rest of her life with leg braces and loss of strength in her hands. Her legal case would finally reach a conclusion, however. The Roberts family eventually settled for medical expenses that totaled nearly $1 million. What most of us do not know is that she also was diagnosed with cancer. She died at the age of seventy in May 2010 following an eleven-year battle with cancer. One cannot make the assumption that her cancer diagnosis resulted from the swine flu vaccine.

However, after researching and finding that out of fifteen people who filed injury claims for the swine flu, five of them died of cancer later in life, a hypothesis can be formulated asking whether there is an increased risk of developing cancer or other major medical diseases or disability as a result of this vaccination. But we might never know the answer to that question. The CDC has whitewashed the swine flu fiasco of 1976. They continue to revise history by publishing papers from the major players in the CDC about "Lessons Learned from the Swine Flu of 1976."

How much money was actually spent on the swine flu fiasco? The initial cost of vaccination had a price tag of $135 million. The actual cost of settling claims could be estimated at $90 million, perhaps double that if Congress ever wanted to audit the program. And add the undetermined cost to Medicaid and Medicare for the expense of providing medical care for those individuals who were not successful in obtaining compensation for their injuries. The bare minimum cost would be $250 million, with estimates closer to $300 to $350 million. In 2014 dollars, the cost would be approximately $1.02 billion to $1.5 billion. The Swine Flu Act of 1976 would serve as a template for Congress in creating the National Vaccine Injury Compensation Program ten years later.

DPT

The vaccine commonly referred to as the DPT is the Diphtheria-Pertussis-Tetanus vaccine. It is often referred to as the "dirty" vaccine and one of the most difficult to manufacture. "Dirty" is meant as a descriptor for a vaccine that has more known side effects than other vaccines.

It was difficult to determine what the adverse reactions were. As infancy is also the time period in which serious medical conditions appeared in both vaccinated and unvaccinated children—seizures, rashes, development delays, SIDS[40]—separating DPT reactions from other illnesses was a very difficult task.[41]

It was the DPT vaccine that would turn the medical community, parents and families, and Congress upside down and lead to the crafting of a national, no-fault vaccine injury compensation program.

It would be the whole-cell pertussis portion of the DPT vaccine that would cause many vaccine-related deaths and severe injuries. And it would be the only vaccine weapon to combat whooping cough, a very serious medical condition that caused many deaths, especially in young children. Nearly seventy-three thousand children died from pertussis from 1922 to 1931, and another 1.7 million cases of whooping cough would be reported during the same time period.

In 1906, Belgian scientist Jules Bordet cultured the bacteria Bordetella pertussis for the first time. There were many attempts to produce a vaccine all the way up to the late 1930s, when Pearl Kendrick and Grace Elderling of the Michigan State Health Department conducted studies of their vaccine, which showed great promise in its efficacy and safety.

In 1940, the pertussis vaccine was combined with the diphtheria and tetanus for the first time. However, seizures and encephalopathy were constant companions to the DPT vaccine. As more monitoring systems were put in place, more reports of vaccine-related injuries were noted. Because of these constant reports of injury, the effort to create a safer vaccine was in the making.

In the mid-1940s, vaccine manufacturer Lederle produced an "extracted" form of the pertussis vaccine. By using a centrifuge, the manufacturer was able to break down the cell walls of the bacteria and extract the liquid. This substance would be more free of the toxins that led to many of the injuries. This was the first known form of acellular pertussis, the vaccine that is used today. However, since this substance used human blood cells as cultured media, it did not pass the Pittman Standard. This was named after Margaret Pittman, who developed a standard for safety and efficacy of testing the pertussis vaccine. Lederle would dump the project. It would be nearly forty more years before a safer form of the pertussis vaccine would be developed, mainly because the pertussis vaccine was so cheap to produce. With a cost of close to a nickel per dose, the manufacturers were not interested in researching and producing a newer or costlier vaccine—until the lawsuits came filing in at courthouses around the country.

In 1975, Charles Manclark, who was hired by the FDA to develop a safer pertussis vaccine, stated the following: "We may be approaching a time in which more vaccine-related problems than those due to the disease will be experienced."[42] Throughout the 1970s and 1980s, the number of lawsuits brought against vaccine manufacturers increased dramatically, and manufacturers made large payouts to individuals and families claiming vaccine injury, particularly from the combined diphtheria-pertussis-tetanus (DPT) immunization.[43] In this environment of increasing litigation, mounting legal fees, and large jury rewards, many pharmaceutical companies left the vaccine business.[44] In fact, by the end of 1984, only one US company still manufactured the DPT vaccine, and other vaccines were losing manufacturers as well.[45]

The number of lawsuits filed prior to the creation of the NVICP as a result of DPT vaccine-related injuries is not as staggering as most would think. In 1979, there was one suit filed, increasing to 255 in 1986 before declining to four in 1997.[46] However, the average asking demand for lawsuits filed in 1985 was $26 million.[47] The entire market size in the United States in 1981 was only $2 million.[48]

The price of the DPT and DT vaccines prior to 1982 was under one dollar.[49] However, the price of DPT increased dramatically, reaching $22, with as much as 96 percent of the price comprised of expected litigation costs.[50] The price of the DT vaccine held steady.[51] After the establishment of the NVICP, the price rapidly declined to $7.40, where it remained until the vaccine was removed from the market.

While the lawsuit filings were in their infancy, so were the grass roots organizations and parent-led groups all advocating for safer vaccines. On April 19, 1982, NBC aired a one-hour documentary called *DPT—Vaccine Roulette*. Reporter Lea Thompson hosted the program and interviewed several families regarding pertussis vaccine-related injuries. Ms. Thompson, who would later receive an Emmy for her reporting on this topic, produced a very hard-hitting and controversial news piece about vaccine injury. She highlighted the story of the Resciniti twins, Leo and Anthony, who both were vaccine injured from the DPT vaccine. They were the cousins of Florida Congressman Dan Mica, a democrat. Dan's brother John was a staff worker for Florida Senator Paula Hawkins, the senator who would introduce legislation in 1983 to establish a vaccine compensation program.

The *DPT—Vaccine Roulette* program created a major stir in the medical community, which basically denied vaccine injuries; the pharmaceutical industry, which was feeling the wrath of lawsuits claiming injuries from the DPT vaccine; and certain media, which wrote how dangerous this program was by undermining the confidence in the vaccine industry. Even today, nearly thirty years later, pro-pharma media sources and medical advocates still write about all the negatives of the hour-long documentary.

When the program aired, Jeff Schwartz and his wife Donna were watching. The experience of what had happened to their daughter was explained in the documentary. Their daughter, Julie, who was born in 1981, received her third DPT vaccine in July 1982. She began suffering seizures and was rushed to the emergency room. The doctor denied that the DPT vaccine could have caused it. The doctors were able to control the grand mal seizure with medication. Tragically, Julie would pass two years later due to the seizure disorder.

Jeff contacted the NBC affiliate in Washington, DC, and told the producers "that they were probably going to get a lot of phone calls from parents stating that this is what happened to their children, and if they are interested, here is my contact information. I would like to talk with them."

Also watching was Kathi Williams, a stay-at-home mother to Nathan, an eighteen-month-old boy who had received his second DPT vaccination four days prior to the show. Nathan, who was a very happy child, screamed for eight hours after receiving the vaccination. Then his leg was sore and he limped for two days. After the show aired, Kathi's mother called her and told her to call the TV station and tell them that the vaccine caused injuries to Nathan.

Barbara Loe Fisher watched a replay of the program the next day. In 1980 her son Christian had received his third DPT vaccine. She recalled that she walked into his room and found him staring at the ceiling. She tried to talk to him but he remained in a foggy state for nearly twenty-four hours. At first she thought that the DPT vaccine had overwhelmed his immune system, although the symptoms that she described were typical of an occasional reaction to the DPT vaccine, according to several safety studies. Later he became sick and started to regress. It wasn't until Barbara Loe Fisher watched the program that she linked her son's medical condition to the DPT vaccine.

When the parents called the TV stations to thank them for airing the program, the producers gave them other parents' contact information. A network of parents was formed as a result of this program. Barbara Loe Fisher and Kathi Williams met informally and started talking about forming a parent's organization focused on vaccine safety. They used the acronym DPT for the name of their parent-led group, Dissatisfied Parents Together.

Jeff Schwartz joined this group, and they met nine days later in the congressional offices of Dan Mica, the congressman from Florida whose twin cousins were featured in the DPT vaccine documentary. Jeff and the congressman knew each other very well, both serving together as staff members for former Congressman Paul Rogers, chairman of the House Commerce Health subcommittee. The documentary would ultimately mobilize a parent-led movement, change the laws, and expose US vaccine policies and systemic questioning for the first time in nearly a century.[52]

It would be this parent movement that would meet with the American Academy of Pediatrics to begin discussions and formulate a framework for creating a vaccine injury compensation program. The parent group did not have compensation as its high priority, but rather wanted safer vaccines, a greater awareness among pediatricians regarding the adverse reactions and risks of the DPT vaccine, and also to ensure that parents have a choice as to whether to administer this vaccine to their children instead of having it be mandatory. The group also wanted the ability for parents to file lawsuits if needed.

Jeff Schwartz, veteran of working in Congress on the Clean Air Act, understood that compromise would be the only way to achieve these goals. The no-fault compensation program being advocated by the Academy of Pediatrics would be a compromise for the parent group. They were still more interested in pursuing or allowing lawsuits to go forth. However, if the compensation program worked well, they agreed that parents would migrate toward that solution. The compromise language that was agreed to by the Academy and the DPT organization would be the basis for what Senator Hawkins from Florida would introduce in 1983. The Reagan Administration wanted no compensation program at all and wanted to terminate all vaccination lawsuits.

Congress felt compelled to address the possibility of a shortage in vaccines but didn't want to respond in a manner that would replicate the Swine Flu Act. Instead, with heavy lobbying by organizations that represented injured parties and vaccine manufacturers, Congress created a no-fault compensation program funded solely by an excise tax on each childhood vaccine. Thus, the Vaccine Act was born from the need to achieve a delicate balance: to support a particular industry by protecting it from civil liability while ensuring that the victims would receive compensation in an expeditious manner.[53]

Chapter 2

Congress and the Vaccine Injury Compensation Program

Because of the lack of success with the Swine Flu Act of 1976, and with US vaccine manufacturers threatening to stop production of vaccines unless they were granted liability protection, Congress proposed legislation that would ultimately shift the liability away from vaccine manufacturers by creating a federally established vaccine injury trust fund and by establishing a specialized no-fault compensation program with a unique court system to adjudicate all claims.

The American Academy of Pediatrics and the parent organization DPT created the basic framework language. Senator Hawkins of Florida agreed to introduce the language, which she did in the 98th Congress, on November 17, 1983, as Senate bill 2117.

The legislation had no provisions to handle off-table causation and injuries. Matter of fact, off-table injuries would be non-compensable in this act. The Senate debate focused on whether the act should be mandatory or an optional alternative remedy. The act would also establish an Advisory Commission on Childhood Vaccines (ACCV) to advise the HHS Secretary on vaccine-related injury standards, vaccine safety, and supply changes.[1] The legislation would receive only one hearing on May 3, 1984, and would not progress any further.

In June 1984, Congressman Waxman of California introduced H.R. 5810. This legislation would grant sole eligibility in compensation jurisdiction to the US District Court located in Washington, DC.[2] The act would establish the ACCV, with similar responsibilities as outlined in Senator Hawkins's S. 2117 bill from 1983. The act also would establish a compensation trust fund within the US Treasury. It would require the HHS Secretary to 1) create a pediatric vaccine risk study, and 2) make related parent information materials available and require the distribution of these materials by pediatric healthcare providers.[3] This would be the origin of the current VIS material.

The act would also require a congressional report to be prepared within two years, and then every two years thereafter.[4] Congressman Waxman's legislation supporters were able to hold and conduct a hearing in September 1984. At this hearing, many stakeholders in the program came together, including the HHS Secretary, the pharmaceutical industry representatives, the American Medical Association, and parent groups, led by Jeffrey Schwartz, the president of the Dissatisfied Parents Together group.

During the congressional hearing Dr. Brandt, who was testifying on behalf of HHS, was asked by Representative Waxman how to prove cause in fact and whether he favored a system that would only compensate individuals whose injuries could be proven. Dr. Brandt answered:

It may very well be impossible to do that in individual cases, at least certainly over the near-term. And I think . . . One has to rely on secondary bits of evidence regarding cause. For example, one would look at epidemiological data and other kinds of data to establish that at least there is a reasonable probability, and I would have to leave "reasonable" undefined for the moment, that a particular adverse event is associated with the vaccine.[5]

Jeffrey Schwartz, speaking on behalf of the parent groups, argued that the three methods most important in separating "cause from coincidence" are 1) the temporal proximity between vaccination and reaction; 2) whether the injuries are consistent with the type of vaccine administered; and 3) whether "an alternative explanation exists that is more persuasive."[6]

As ambitious as this legislation was, it did not have the necessary votes to pass in Congress. However, Congress was not done, and for each attempt to pass legislation, more components would be advanced.

In March 1985, Representative Madigan of Illinois introduced HR 1780. This legislation would prohibit the filing of the civil tort action for damages unless the procedures of the act had been followed.[7] The act would also set aggregate limits for damages of vaccine-related injuries to $1 million, including $100,000 for pain and suffering.[8] One of the more troubling components of this legislation would require the HHS Secretary to establish "hearing panels" to determine the validity of each petition that was submitted.[9] Thus, the hearing panel would be empowered to determine whether any alleged injuries or deaths were vaccine-related and, if appropriate, to award compensation.[10] Also, the first mention of the statute of limitations was included in this legislation and declared that all claims filed more than two years after the first manifestation of a vaccine-related injury would be barred.

The act also established the ACCV to 1) advise the HHS Secretary on the implementation of the program; 2) study and recommend ways to encourage the availability of safe and effective vaccines; 3) survey information-gathering programs and advise the secretary of how to obtain useful information; and 4) recommend research.[11]

Senator Hawkins of Florida again introduced legislation, this time in April 1985, with S827, known as the National Childhood Vaccine Improvement Act of 1986. The act would require the ACCV to conduct certain studies, including 1) assuring the availability of safe and effective childhood vaccines; 2) examining the relationship between vaccines containing pertussis and Reye syndrome, sudden infant death syndrome, juvenile diabetes, and other diseases; and 3) looking at children associated with each childhood vaccine.[12]

The act would also require healthcare providers who administer a childhood vaccine to record certain information with respect to each vaccine and with respect to resulting complications of immunizations. The act would require healthcare providers and vaccine manufacturers to report certain information to the HHS Secretary. Thus were the beginnings of the current Vaccine Adverse Event Reporting System, or VAERS. The act also directed the HHS Secretary to conduct research to identify and develop a safe pertussis vaccine.[13]

A few months later, on September 18, 1986, Representative Waxman introduced HR 5546, which would eventually become the National Childhood Vaccine Injury Act of 1986.[14] This is the bill that President Ronald Reagan signed into law on November 14, 1986, with some "mixed feelings."[15] President Reagan had reservations about a compensation program that allowed people to obtain payments or compensation from the federal government without proving fault or wrongdoing by the vaccine manufacturer.[16] The bill was part of a much larger Omnibus Health Bill (S.1744). The White House floated the idea of vetoing the entire omnibus package mainly because of the NCVIA. However, Vice President George

H. W. Bush and Secretary of the Treasury James Baker motivated President Reagan to sign the bill into law.[17]

The act borrowed several components of previous legislation attempts, such as requiring petitioners to file a claim in the program prior to seeking civil tort action in state or federal court. The act also provided "no liability" to vaccine manufacturers and established the National Vaccine Injury Compensation Program as an alternative remedy to judicial action for vaccine-related injuries.[18] The act also granted the US District Court system the authority to determine eligibility for compensation. It set forth the table of injuries deemed vaccine-related for compensation purposes.[19]

The act permitted the Secretary of Health and Human Services to establish guidelines to revise the Vaccine Injury Table (VIT) and to recommend changes to the vaccines covered by the table.[20] The parent group DPT had concerns about the HHS Secretary having the ability to modify the vaccine injury table. They would ultimately agree to allow the secretary to make those changes but with judicial oversight; however, that provision did not make it into the final bill. Thus the Secretary of the HHS has the ultimate ability to modify the vaccine injury table without congressional or judicial oversight.

The Department of Health and Human Services (HHS) along with the Department of Justice (DOJ) opposed all efforts to create a compensation program from the very beginning.[21] The act granted them rulemaking authority, thus giving them most of the power to revise or change everything after the law was passed.[22]

The act also specified that compensation awards under the program shall be paid out of the Vaccine Injury Trust Fund with limits up to $250,000 for pain and suffering and up to $250,000 for death, and also prohibited compensation for punitive damages. It established the ACCV to 1) advise the secretary on implementation of the program; 2) recommend changes to the vaccine injury table; and 3) recommend research priorities.

The act further continued by 1) requiring the secretary to develop certain vaccine information materials for distribution to parents or legal representatives of anyone receiving a vaccine listed in the injury table; and 2) directing the Secretary to promote the development of safer childhood vaccines.[23]

But one of the most overlooked provisions of the act was the requirement that the HHS Secretary conduct public awareness and outreach programs to inform the general public about the program and the eligibility to file a claim for either a vaccine-related injury or death. (In § 300aa-10. Establishment of Program, (c) Publicity. The Secretary shall undertake reasonable efforts to inform the public of the availability of the program.)

This provision has been greatly ignored by the HHS Secretary. Later in this book I will outline the failed attempts by the Secretary in this area. There was no guidance or direction offered by the act for the court to adjudicate off-table vaccine-related injuries or death. This oversight would lead to great inconsistency in how the court would interpret off-table injuries and would be very punitive toward the petitioner.

Chapter 3

Congressional Oversight

As quickly as Congress passed legislation at the end of 1986, the congressional oversight of the same program disappeared. It would be thirteen years before Congress, via congressional hearings or by the United States General Accounting Office (GAO), would be informed of the progress of the NVICP. A GAO report was presented to Congress in December 1999 entitled "Vaccine Injury Compensation: Program Challenged to Settle Claims Quickly and Easily." The office of the GAO is required by law to review trust funds and their adequacy to meet future claims.[1]

In this GAO report, most of the emphasis was placed upon the court's ability to settle claims in an efficient and quick manner. The intention of Congress was to have an average length of time for most claims to be decided within one year. That average quickly rose to two years and higher, and during the early 1990s many claims took three to five years, with several taking longer. All claims of vaccine-related injury or death that occurred prior to the establishment of the program had to be filed by January 31, 1991. And with the addition of Hepatitis B vaccine to the program, with a filing deadline of August 1999 and the "grandfathering" of all claims going back eight years, a large backlog of petitions ensued, only to slow down the adjudication process further.

The GAO report noted that 4,245 claims were filed as a result of vaccines administered to persons prior to October 1, 1988.[2] These claims, sometimes known as "pre-act" petitions, accounted for nearly $745,000,000 in compensable awards and petitioner attorney fees.[3] The funding source for all awards was the US General Fund. All compensable awards and petitioner attorney fees for claims as the result of vaccines administered on or after October 1, 1988 were funded by the newly established Vaccine Injury Trust Fund. The source for the trust fund was the $0.75 excise tax on each antigen component of a vaccine dose sold. The measles, mumps, and rubella (MMR) vaccine, as an example, would contribute $2.25 in excise taxes to the trust fund.

When the GAO report looked into the reasons behind why the time to adjudicate claims increased dramatically beyond what Congress had in mind, they noted one area that many parent groups and advocates had been talking about for many years. When Congress created the NVICP, they transferred complete rulemaking authority to the HHS Secretary to change the Vaccine Injury Table.

In testimony on September 28, 1999, to the House Subcommittee on Criminal Justice, Drug Policy, and Human Resources, Barbara Loe Fisher, one of the key parent advocates and architects of the original legislation to establish the NVICP, stated the following:

> The principal reason why the Vaccine Injury Compensation Program has become highly adversarial and is turning away three out of four claimants is that the Department of Health and Human Services (DHHS), with the assistance of the Department of Justice (DOJ), has wielded its discretionary authority to all but eliminate a just list of compensable events

in the Vaccine Injury Table, thereby destroying the guiding tenet of presumption. This action by DHHS constitutes the most egregious violation of the spirit and intent of the law and, in effect, is a fatal compromise of its integrity.

Ironically, it was the understanding of parents who participated in the development of the law that Congress granted the HHS Secretary broad discretionary authority to alter the Vaccine Injury Table primarily so the secretary could expand the list of compensable events and make the system more inclusive, not less inclusive. It was understood that the intent was to provide the secretary with flexibility to accommodate the addition of new presumptions for injuries associated with the administration of existing and future vaccines.

However, over time, the secretary has primarily used her discretionary authority through the regulatory process to remove compensable events from the table sanctioned by Congress and to refine permanent injuries in the Aids to Interpretation long recognized by the medical community as being associated with vaccine reactions. In the words of one attorney for vaccine-injured children, the secretary's arbitrary redefinition of the medically recognized definition of "encephalopathy" is so restrictive that it is believed by petitioners' counsels across this country that they will never again see an injury to a child that falls within the definition's narrow confines.[4]

Most of the contention surrounding the changes to the Vaccine Injury Table (VIT) focused on the changes done in 1995 and 1997 by then HHS Secretary Donna Shalala. One major change was removing Residual Seizure Disorder (RSD) from the table. In 1995, RSD was removed from the table relating to pertussis and tetanus vaccines. In 1997, RSD was removed from the table relating to the MMR vaccine.

The other major change to the VIT was the arbitrary revision of the encephalopathy definition (brain injury). The secretary, using her rulemaking authority, acted upon the Institute of Medicine's (IOM) report stating that they found the evidence inadequate to accept or reject a causal relationship between vaccine and residual disorder.[5] In addition, the nine vaccines added to the table by the HHS Secretary since 1988 generally have no specific table injuries at all or have the immediate onset of anaphylactic shock as the only listed table injury.[6] This alone guarantees that most petitions filed in the program today are off-table injuries, ensuring a very litigious environment for petitioners.

The office of the HHS Secretary published its reasoning for each revision to the Vaccine Injury Table in the Federal Register but has not published an overall method of applying the criteria it uses in conjunction with the IOM findings.[7] For table changes, the secretary is only required to provide a 180-day public notice and comment period and a ninety-day review period for the ACCV.[8]

HHS often interprets the intent of Congress and its own rulemaking authority by recognizing table injuries where there are definitive studies or research linking vaccines to the table injuries. Parent advocates and others would interpret the rulemaking authority granted to HHS as directing the secretary as to the idea that until definitive data is available, the benefit of the doubt should remain with the petitioner.

Thus, the decision by the secretary, which interpreted the inconclusive data report from IOM on Residual Seizure Disorder as "definitive" proof that no causal relationship existed, has come under great scrutiny.

The IOM's recommendations to the HHS Secretary should be considered arbitrary at best. For example, the IOM found that existing scientific evidence favored acceptance of a causal relationship between tetanus vaccines and brachial neuritis, and the HHS Secretary added this to the Vaccine Injury Table.[9] On the other hand, the IOM found a similar relationship between the tetanus and polio vaccine and Guillain-Barré Syndrome (GBS). The HHS Secretary did not add this to the table.[10]

The IOM found the evidence inadequate to accept or reject a causal relationship between vaccines and Residual Seizure Disorder and thus the HHS Secretary removed this condition from the table.[11] The same finding of the MMR and encephalopathy remained in the table.[12]

The secretary has yet to create a Vaccine Injury Table for the Trivalent Influenza vaccine and the newly approved Quadrivalent Influenza vaccine. During the December 2013 quarterly meeting, the ACCV approved a new addition to the Vaccine Injury Table for the influenza vaccines: Guillain-Barré Syndrome.[13] The secretary has yet to act upon the approval from the ACCV and make that addition to the table. The overwhelming majority of petitions filed in the program over the last two to three years deal with injuries as a result of the influenza vaccination. And the majority of those injuries are Guillain-Barré Syndrome.

The Department of Health and Human Services' own inspector general issued a report to the secretary, nearly seven years before the GAO report, heavily criticizing the manner in which the program handled the large number of petitions filed and how those petitions were decided. In his report, the inspector general noted the following: "a review of all completed cases, as of August 1991, reveals that 58 percent of the cases that the HHS internal medical staff recommended not be compensated were overturned by the special masters and compensated."[14] The report continues by citing two major factors that account for the reversal rate: 1) lack of corroboration of evidence and 2) various interpretations of the Vaccine Injury Table.[15]

The current balance of the vaccine trust fund, as of early 2014, is approximately $3.42 billion. Since its inception, the trust fund has received more in vaccine excise taxes than it has paid out for compensable damages, attorney fees, and administrative costs. The current excise tax of $0.75 per dose has been commonly reported as income to the trust fund. However, that is not the case. Since the program began, the US Treasury collects the excise tax from the vaccine manufacturers and transfers that tax, less a 25 percent offset, to the vaccine injury trust fund.[16] As provided in section 9602(b) of the Internal Revenue Code for management of trust funds in general, the US General Fund has been receiving $.19 out of the $.75 excise tax for every dose sold.[17] Thus, the trust fund only receives $.56 instead of the publicly promoted $.75 levy. But our federal government is not done raiding the fund.

Each year, Congress appropriates money out of the trust fund and directs it to HHS, DOJ, and the court for their administration of the program. Health Resources and Service Administration (HRSA), a division of HHS, receives the largest appropriation out of the trust fund mainly due to their responsibility of paying out compensable damages and attorney fees. However, the difference between those outlays and the total appropriation from the fund has been increasing dramatically over the last decade. The same could be said of DOJ and the court. Some of the compensation is directed toward salaries, wages, and administrative costs of the program. However, suspicion is raised when examining the monthly and yearly trust fund budget reports, as published on the US Treasury website.[18]

Per the GAO report of March 2000 to Congress regarding the Vaccine Injury Trust Fund, "current annual appropriation levels to reimburse agencies from the VIT for administrative expenses—about $9.6 million—appear sufficient to meet agency needs."[19] HHS administers the program, with involvement by the Department of Justice and the US Court of Federal Claims to help adjudicate injury claims.[20] In earlier years of the program, administrative expenses incurred by these agencies sometimes exceeded the amounts appropriated from the trust fund to reimburse them.[21] From fiscal year 1996 through the end of fiscal year 1999, the trust fund appropriation was increased from about $7.8 million to $9.4

million, appropriated amounts having exceeded actual expenses by 3 to 11 percent each year.[22]

An untrained eye examining the balance sheet reports of the vaccine trust fund for the recent fiscal years will find that HRSA, DOJ, and the court are increasing their appropriation for administration of the program. It would be wise for the GAO to examine these appropriations, especially in light of the current federal budget concerns around sequester and budget cuts. The trust fund is not a bank to help balance these agencies' budgets.

DOJ officials have refused to respond to Freedom of Information Act (FOIA) requests by this author regarding how much money is being spent per petition on DOJ attorney fees, outside contracted medical expert fees and costs, and internal medical review, by stating that this information is legal privilege and would disclose their legal strategy in prosecuting claims in the program. The general public is informed of the compensable damage awards and related attorney fees and costs for each petition as part of the final decision of each petition.

HRSA officials have refused to respond to FOIA requests by this author regarding contracts, documents, and funding of IOM reports used by the HHS Secretary to advise on potential changes to the table and DOJ attorneys prosecuting petitions in the program. There have been suspicions raised by members of the Advisory Commission on Childhood Vaccines that the VIT was the ultimate payer of these research studies. This could be interpreted as a violation of current federal law, since the VIT was not established to fund vaccine research studies.

Because of the ever-increasing balance of the VIT, the ongoing discussion and debate regarding it has brought vaccine manufacturers, officials from HHS, the FDA, and the CDC, along with parent advocate groups together in proposing options to address the large trust fund balance. Most of the discussion has involved cutting the excise tax that supports the trust fund or spending more of the money received on designated vaccine-related activities.[23]

Some of the vaccine manufacturers view the trust fund balance as too high and want to reduce the excise tax. This will meet some considerable resistance from Congress because of the decreased revenue generation to the US General Fund and from parent advocates who helped craft the original legislation. HHS, FDA, and CDC officials see the high balance of the trust fund as a potential revenue source if Congress decides to expand trust fund spending to vaccine-related activities such as providing funding for vaccine injury surveillance systems or for research examining links between vaccines and injuries or diseases.[24]

Parent advocates, some members of Congress, and attorneys representing petitioners in the program, seeing the ever-increasing balance of the trust fund, called on Congress to reestablish the Vaccine Injury Table back to its original intentions. They are also asking for an increase in the existing cap limits for pain-and-suffering and the death benefit from $250,000, increasing the allowable reimbursement rates for medical experts testifying on the behalf of petitioners, and expediting the reimbursements to the petitioner's medical experts. This will allow a more equitable and compassionate compensation program for those who were injured by vaccines.

Congress needs to request meaningful GAO audit reports of the program itself and also order audits of the Vaccine Injury Trust Fund on a more frequent basis. As one attorney who practices in the program told me, the trust fund has turned into a personal piggy bank for a couple of government agencies. There is a high probability that far more money is being spent on administration and management of the NVICP and trust fund than on the compensation of vaccine-related-injury petitioners.

Chapter 4

De Minimis

The Vaccine Act of 1986 created a process to allow individuals seeking compensation for vaccine-related injury or death to file a petition with the NVICP. In the early years of the program, a requirement for filing a petition required the petitioner to meet what has become commonly known as the severity clause. This clause requires an individual to display residual effects of their vaccine injury for at least six months and also to have incurred unreimbursed medical expenses of at least $1,000. And in the cases of death, the petitioner/representative of the estate of the deceased must prove that the death was the result of the vaccine. These requirements are intended to bar compensation for *de minimis*, or minor, injuries.

These requirements were inserted into the statute by Congress to prevent petition filings for minor injuries. The $1,000 requirement came under great scrutiny during the 1990s as many petitions were automatically dismissed because of the lack of providing documents or receipts for unreimbursed medical expenses. These petitions were not judged on the merits of the injury or injuries but rather the inability to provide documentation for costs incurred.

One such petition that was dismissed involves an American Indian boy by the name of Daniel Black. His petition was dismissed because his medical expenses at the time were covered by Indian Health Services. His injury, which was severe, could not be addressed in the NVICP because of the lack of unreimbursed medical expenses. The Indian Health Services paid all of his initial medical expenses, which totaled over $17,000. Thus, young Daniel Black was never able to present his case.

Natalie Rodriguez, another victim of the hard statutes of the program, suffered a vaccine-related injury from her fourth DPT vaccination, which was administered to her in October 1984. The petition included medical records stating that she suffered from a seizure disorder, which is a table injury. This petition clearly should be awarded compensation. However, Natalie and her parents have Medicaid instead of private insurance. Therefore, she did not meet the $1,000 in unreimbursed expenses mandate. The special master had to dismiss the petition on the grounds of failure to present a *prima facie* case. Thus, another child is vaccine injured and is denied compensation due to Medicaid coverage. And if the child were born to military parents as well, or someone with low-deductible insurance plans, would this be the case, as well? Is this what Congress intended? Ironically, if those persons under Medicaid could muster the $1,000 in order to come under the program, their compensation under the act would eliminate Medicaid as a payer of their medical expenses.

The second part of the severity clause states that an individual who files a petition must display residual effects of that vaccine injury for at least six months. A cursory reading of the statute regarding the six-month requirement can be justified as reasonable. As enforced as policy, however, it is not without its problems, lacks fairness, and in certain situations is indefensible. Congress or the courts need to review the statute especially as it pertains to young children. Later in this chapter I will present to you the story of a two-year-old boy, G. S., whose petition was dismissed because he did not suffer the residual effects of his vaccine and associated injury for more than six months.

To better understand the discussion and debate surrounding the six-month injury requirement of the act, a re-examination of the rotavirus vaccine and the actions of the Centers for Disease Control and Prevention (CDC) and its Advisory Committee on Immunization Practices (ACIP) recommending the vaccine for routine administration to infants must be discussed.

In March 1999, ACIP recommended the rotavirus vaccine for routine administration to infants in the United States. In July 1999, all vaccines against rotavirus were added to the vaccine injury table without specific associated table injuries. Later, in November 1999, after reviewing scientific data, including reports to the Vaccine Adverse Events Reporting System (VAERS) of intussusception among fifteen infants who received the rotavirus vaccine, the ACIP withdrew its recommendation.

Following ACIP's recommendation, a bill to amend the Vaccine Act was proposed in the United States Senate. One of the bill's sponsors noted, however, that a new situation developed that was not foreseeable at the time of enactment of this law in 1986. Some cases of intussusception required hospitalization and surgery, and under the law as it stood then, such cases would not be compensated. Thus, the bill sponsors proposed that subsection 11(c)(1)(D) be amended to include patients who "suffered such illness, disability, injury or condition from the vaccine which resulted in inpatient hospitalization and surgical intervention to correct such illness, disability, injury or condition."[1] This amendment would only apply to circumstances under which a vaccine recipient suffered from intussusception as a result of the administration of the rotavirus vaccine, and not from other vaccines and their associated injuries.

In September 2000, the bill to amend subsection 11(c)(1)(D) was passed by the House of Representatives. In true Washington, DC. form, the congressional record does not reflect any debate concerning the proposed amendment; there was no discussion of restricting the amendment injuries due only to the rotavirus vaccine. The actual language of the amendment as passed does not contain any such restriction. However, the clause "to correct such illness, disability, injury or condition" was omitted from the final version of the amendment.

Currently, to be eligible for an award of vaccine compensation, a petitioner must prove by a preponderance of the evidence that the petitioner suffered vaccine-related injury meeting one of three severity requirements:

A. suffered the residual effects or complications of such illness, disability, injury, or condition for more than six months after the ministration of the vaccine,[2] or

B. died from the administration of the vaccine,[3] or

C. suffered such illness, disability, injury, or condition from the vaccine that resulted in inpatient hospitalization and surgical intervention.[4]

The last two words from part C regarding the severity clause still needs to be addressed either by Congress or the Federal Circuit Court of Appeals. The term "surgical intervention" is not defined in the act. Consequently, the special master will have to make that determination on a case-by-case basis. In the case of *G. S. v. HHS*, the special master ruled that the IV therapy does not qualify as a "surgical intervention." Thus, according to the special master's interpretation, the petitioner has failed to present factual evidence that G. S. suffered an injury that satisfies the vaccine act's severity requirement. And the respondent's motion to dismiss is granted.

The Vaccine Act's six-month injury requirement prevents many petitioners from receiving compensation. Prior to the year 2000, petitioners claiming that the rotavirus vaccine caused their child's intussusception were denied compensation. Since most patients with intussusception recovered after immediate treatment and did not suffer lasting complications for more than six months, those petitioners alleging intussusception would have been denied compensation under the pre–year 2000 amendment standard.[5]

In 2000, however, the act was amended in response to the discovery of a connection between the rotavirus vaccine and intussusception. Congressional sponsors of the legislation to amend the act stated that in some cases intussusception required hospitalization and surgery, and under the laws it stood then that such cases would not be compensated.

Daniel Black v. HHS

The story of Daniel Black, an American Indian child, began when he received a DPT vaccination in December 1984 at an Indian Health Services hospital. Daniel developed serious medical problems within a few days as a result of an adverse reaction to the DPT vaccine.

The Vaccine Act of 1986 provided a filing deadline for those who were injured or have died as a result of a vaccine administered prior to the establishment of the program. The initial deadline was October 1, 1990. The HHS Secretary extended the filing period to January 31, 1991.

On October 1, 1990, Daniel's father filed a petition on his behalf, seeking compensation for injuries incurred from the DPT vaccination in December 1984. In the petition, medical records were submitted that noted that within hours of receiving the DPT vaccine, Daniel suffered a seizure. He continued to suffer severe seizure episodes throughout his infancy.

As a result of the DPT vaccine and subsequent seizure episodes, Daniel developed profound impairments and experienced severe developmental delays. In a paper published in August 1997 in the *American University Law Review*, Daniel's attorney, James Leach, stated that "Daniel is suffering from serious learning disabilities that include visual perceptual deficits and auditory comprehension deficits, as well as short- and long-term memory problems. He has severe problems with attention and concentration, displaying restlessness and high levels of distractibility that result in a poor ability to attend to matters at hand. He is the lowest functioning child in the classroom of emotional and behavioral disturbed and learning disabled children."[6]

Mr. Leach continued, "Daniel's school does not have the resources to provide adequate speech or occupational therapy. He functions in a borderline range of tested intelligence, his daily skills and behaviors even lower due to perceptual and auditory problems, as well as his attention deficit and hyperactivity disorder. He is delayed in language development and fine motor skills. He is socially immature, aggressive, and difficult to manage. Intensive therapy is necessary to control his behavior. When he becomes an adult, Daniel will be unable to live independently. He will need to be in a supervised living setting providing behavioral programming. He may be able to work in a supported employment program. Because Daniel's petition was dismissed and excluded, he will not receive compensation equipment, residential and custodial care and services, and related travel facilities expenses. Nor will he receive compensation for projected lifetime loss of earnings, for actual and projected pain-and-suffering, or for emotional distress."[7]

Daniel's attorney appealed the decision by the special master to dismiss the petition. In their decision to affirm the special master's ruling for dismissal, the court held that the Indian Health Services payments for Daniel's medical expenses excluded him because "the $1,000.00 in expenses is a threshold criterion for seeking entry into the compensation program. In order to file a valid petition, the injured person must have incurred at least $1,000.00 in unreimbursable expenses."

After the dismissal of his petition, his attorney fought feverishly to have the decision reviewed and then later appealed. Mr. Leach argued on behalf of his client, Daniel Black, "that there is no guarantee of continued health care benefits because he is Native American. The Indian Health Services is perennially underfunded. Future funding is subject to shifting political winds and hard economic realities as the federal government continues to downsize. The Indian Health Service decision to discontinue any healthcare program is committed to its discretion and is not subject to judicial review."

A Federal Court of Claims judge dismissed the motion for review and the Federal Circuit Court of Appeals affirmed the special master's decision. Mr. Leach concluded in his argument that "Native Americans should not suffer because of their race by being denied the benefits of the vaccine act compensation for their injuries."[8]

The attorney outlined his case that Daniel Black should have had his petition judged in the NVICP and wrote the paper mentioned earlier, published in the *American University Law Review*. In this paper, Mr. Leach stated the following: "Congress should amend the vaccine act so that other profoundly injured Native American vaccine victims like Daniel Black are not denied lifetime compensation merely because the Indian Health Services paid their initial medical expenses."[9]

Continuing to fight for his client, the attorney reached out to US Senator Tom Daschle of South Dakota and presented his case on why the Vaccine Act of 1986 unintentionally created a burden that was too high for certain petitioners. Federal courts had previously upheld the constitutionality of this requirement under the Fifth Amendment Equal Protection Clause, since "as a general matter, those who incur only modest expenses or whose expenses are reimbursed from other sources present less compelling cases for compensation than those who incur large, unreimbursed expenses."[10] In the fall of 1998, the Reconciliation Budget bill included language to amend the act by eliminating the $1,000.00 unreimbursed medical expenses requirement.

So what about Daniel Black? Currently, he requires around-the-clock medical care for his injuries. His family has incurred thousands of dollars of expenses after his petition to provide appropriate medical care for their son was dismissed. Now imagine if this requirement did not exist prior to the filing of Black's petition. And how many other injured children did this affect? That is difficult to determine but worthy of ongoing research.

Would *Daniel Black v. HHS* proceed further in the program and ultimately win compensation? A review of his petition would lead one to believe that he would have been successful. However, we will never know; his petition was dismissed and is now time-barred.

G. S. v. HHS

In March 2010, G. S. received a hepatitis A vaccine at his two-year well-baby checkup. Five days later, the boy's mother and G. S. returned to the pediatrician reporting that he was "off balance trying to walk" recently. A couple days later, G. S. returned to the pediatrician's office yet again and his mother told the doctor that he was still weak, was falling down a lot, and could not get back up.

Later that day, G. S. was admitted to the hospital and a neurologic exam found him to be "notable for mild lower extremity, decreased tone and areflexia, the absent of reflexes, and there was concern for GBS."

The following day the young boy underwent a lumbar puncture commonly known as a spinal tap. This procedure is essential in confirming the diagnosis of conditions including meningitis and encephalitis, and helpful in diagnosing demyelinating diseases. For those who know about the spinal tap procedure, it can be painful and unnerving for the parents—and dangerous. However it is noted by the doctors that with proper sedation and local anesthesia, a spinal tap should not be overly distressing or painful to most patients.

In addition to the lumbar puncture, the young boy also received two days of IV treatments. G. S. was discharged three days later and, according to his doctors, his condition had improved. Five months later, the boy's mother reported back to the pediatrician that her son was back to his prior behaviors and did not exhibit any after effects of his hospitalization and treatment.

In her petition filed with the NVICP, G. S.'s mother claimed that the hepatitis A vaccine caused her child to suffer Guillain-Barré Syndrome. The respondent filed a motion to dismiss the petition because the injured party failed to satisfy the vaccine act's severity requirement. Specifically, the respondent asserts that the child did not suffer the residual effects or complications of such illness, disability, injury, or condition for more than six months after the administration of the vaccine and did not suffer a vaccine injury resulting in surgical intervention.[11] The special master granted the respondent's motion to dismiss.

In their motion to dismiss, the respondent asserted that a lumbar puncture is a medical and diagnostic procedure, not a surgical procedure. Additionally, the respondent contended that G. S. "was asymptomatic for five months post-vaccination, and thus did not suffer a vaccine-related injury persisting for more than six months." Petitioner filed a response to the respondent's motion to dismiss arguing that both the lumbar procedure and the IV therapy that G. S. received while hospitalized satisfied the surgical intervention requirement. Regarding the act's six-month injury requirement, the petitioner added that it's inconceivable that G. S. did not suffer at least one month of emotional distress after his ordeal.

So now, what will happen to the young lad, G. S.? Let's pray that no harm has come to him, and that his future will be bright and without any long-term effects of what he had to endure for several months. And this does raise the question of why it is necessary for young children, those in the earliest stages of life, to endure sometimes painful and emotional distress before the NVICP will entertain a petition for compensation. Why were six months selected as the magic number of months to endure the residual effects of injury before one can file a petition?

Chapter 5

Pro Se

West's *Encyclopedia of American Law* defines *pro se* as "for one's own behalf; in person. Appearing for oneself, as in the case of one who does not retain a lawyer and appears for himself or herself in court."

It is an established tenet that you have the right to represent yourself in a court of law. However, many people do not understand that choosing to represent yourself means that the court will expect you to follow the same rules and procedures that an attorney must follow.[1]

Filing a petition in the NVICP *pro se* is an option for families that cannot find an attorney who will represent them. For many of these families, it is the only option as they race against the clock, the three-year statute of limitations for injury, or two-year time frame for their loved ones who died. Some of these families will obtain legal representation after filing the initial petition. But for some, the family will proceed on their own.

The Supreme Court has held that courts must construe the content of *pro se* filings liberally.[2] However, being a *pro se* litigant does not relieve the petitioner of his burden to fulfill the statutory requirements of the Vaccine Act. In my review of the success rate of all *pro se* petitions filed in the NVICP, less than 1 percent have resulted in compensation.

Many cases might be originally filed as *pro se*, thus stopping the clock on the statute of limitations. Then the petitioner has some time to find a qualified attorney to represent their interests.

Also, many attorneys will file motions with the court to terminate their representation of their client due to irreconcilable differences, or if the client wants to be represented by another attorney.

There are a few major reasons to consider not to file as a *pro se* case.

1. It is very difficult to find a medical expert to testify on your behalf. Most medical experts who testify on a regular basis with the court are known to most of the attorneys who represent petitioners. Due to the delay in processing payments for the fees and costs for medical experts, unless the *pro se* petitioner can fund these costs up front, most of the time medical experts are not utilized.

2. Even though the special masters will grant a little more latitude regarding proceedings for a *pro se* petitioner, the demands on the petitioner to obtain and file the necessary medical reports, documents, and other materials as the court requires is taxing, especially for a parent who is trying to provide care to the injured party and at the same time is representing them in the NVICP.

3. As attorneys become more aggressive in their screening process when accepting clients, more and more petitioners will be faced with the reality of going it alone, especially for those cases that are off-table injuries. Some would argue that the court and the Secretary of HHS have forced most petitions filed in the current years to be causation cases, and it is becoming more difficult to fully prosecute this type of case. This creates a barrier that was not envisioned by Congress when they passed the Vaccine Act of 1986.

In "an analysis of the first eight years of the NVICP, there were 786 contested claims resolved through published judicial opinions. The likelihood of compensation depended in part on the closeness of the match between the described injury and a specific list of acknowledged vaccine side effects. In addition, the chances of the petitioner winning compensation were influenced by the petitioner's choice of attorney and expert witnesses, by the assignment of the special master to decide the case, and increasingly over time, by the petitioner's ability to comply with procedural requirements."[3]

The following is the story of Gayle DeLong and her *pro se* representation of her daughter's petition in the NVICP.

DeLong v. HHS

Gayle DeLong and her husband, Jonathan Rose, have two daughters, Jenny and her younger sister, Flora.

Flora was born in January 2000. She was diagnosed with mild PDD-NOS at the age of three and a half. Her doctors told Gayle and Jonathan that this was one of the mildest cases of autism that the doctor had ever seen.

Flora became slowly but steadily worse during 2004. Then, she had a precipitous drop in 2005 after receiving her MMR booster at the age of five in January of that year. This began the difficult and heartbreaking journey as her autism became more pronounced and more debilitating.

Her older sister, Jenny, also suffers from autism and responds to Applied Behavioral Analysis (ABA) up to a point. At first, Gayle and Jonathan did not suspect Flora was vaccine injured. Even when Gayle's neighbor confessed to them that she heard Don Imus talk about vaccine problems, Gayle rejected the vaccine link for Flora.

Her father-in-law suggested that Gayle and Jonathan read David Kirby's groundbreaking book, *Evidence of Harm*. Jonathan was the first to read the book and concluded quickly that Flora was vaccine injured, possibly by mercury. Gayle immediately started calling DAN! (Defeat Autism Now) doctors in their area, looking for solutions to help treat Flora and Jenny.

On May 5, 2005, while the rest of the nation was celebrating Cinco de Mayo, Gayle filled out the new patient forms so her girls could see a DAN! doctor whose office was an hour away from their home. As Gayle started to learn about vaccine injuries, she felt betrayed by the country she loved so much. She thought, *How can our government promote a vaccine schedule that is damaging to children?*

Later in 2005, she started to think about filing a claim or petition with the National Vaccine Injury Compensation Program to seek compensation for Flora's injury. Gayle and Jonathan suspected Jenny was vaccine injured as well, but as they found out later, it was too late to file a claim with the court due to the short three-year filing period.

A friend of Gayle's mentioned that she had already filed a petition and recommended Kevin Conway and Ronald Homer of Conway, Homer & Chin-Caplin, P.C., a law firm from Boston that specialized in vaccine-injury cases.

Gayle contacted the law firm immediately and was told that the firm was not accepting any more thimerosal cases since thimerosal was removed from the vaccine schedule several years before. They did send her the short form to file on her own, *pro-se.*

The initial petition was filed March 27, 2006. Since the parents felt the injury was first apparent only when the diagnosis of autism was made, they thought they were in compliance with the three-year statute of limitations, from the date of injury to the filing date.

A month later, a notice was sent from the court to the parents regarding the case filing and consideration for the Omnibus Autism Proceedings by the current special master assigned to her case, George Hastings. It was nearly a year later that a new special master, Denise Vowell, would be assigned to the case.

Two years passed. A court order dated February 13, 2009, a formality, was sent to the family requesting all medical records. Petitioners have ninety days to comply with this order. This process was exhaustive and time-consuming. Gayle needed a sixty-day extension to file stage 1 medical records, which she applied for and received in May 2009. Since she did not work in the summer, she was able to devote a major amount of time in June to compiling the requested papers. She filed the papers in July. Two months later, she received notice that the court had received them.

As Congress stated in the passage of the NVICP legislation, the intent was to provide a quick, non-adversarial forum for petitioners to file claims. Three years passed since the filing of the petition with the court and still no resolution. So much for being quick.

In October 2009, a motion was filed by the respondent, the Secretary of Health and Human Services, to dismiss the claim.

Nearly a year later, in September 2010, Gayle received a notice from the court requiring her "to provide, within 90 days of that order, a reliable medical expert's opinion to establish (1) a medical theory causally connecting the vaccination to the injury; (2) a logical sequence of the cause and effect showing the vaccination was the reason for the injury; and (3) a showing of a proximate temporal relationship between the vaccination and the injury."

The order continued by stating, "You must inform the court within thirty days of the date of this order how you wish to proceed. If you inform the court that you wish to continue to pursue your claim, you will receive another order directing you to file the medical expert's opinion and other evidence necessary to decide your claim. Failure to file a timely response to this order will lead to dismissal of your claim."

This notice and order from the court can be intimidating to parents who are dealing with their vaccine-injured child, seeking appropriate medical care, more often than not fighting their schools regarding educational services, and trying to keep gainful employment for their family.

One of the most difficult items to comply with is to find a medical expert who will provide testimony and documentation as to the injury in question. It is not that there is not enough evidence; it is a fact of finding a medical expert who will come forward without the threat of retribution or other sanctions being filed against that medical practitioner.

In October 2010, four and a half years since the filing, Gayle filed a response to pursue a claim. A couple of days later, the court ordered Gayle to "provide the court within thirty days of the date of this order a statement identifying petitioner's theory regarding the vaccine's relationship to Petitioner's Injury. Failure to file a timely Response to this Order will lead to dismissal of your claim."

Throughout this entire process, Gayle had become more pessimistic about the Vaccine Court doing what was right and just. And from a bystander's viewpoint, the Vaccine Court had morphed into a very adversarial environment, intimidating all who enter the program. "This case was so emotionally draining, especially the first couple of years," said Gayle.

Nine months passed, and it was August 2011 before the court acted again, this time to review the findings of *Cloer v. HHS,* a recent decision by the US Court of Appeals for the Federal Circuit. *Cloer v. HHS* is a case regarding a decision on the three-year statute of limitations to file a claim. Remember that at the beginning of this case, the parents were not at all certain that their daughter had autism until she received a diagnosis—"one of the mildest the doctor had ever seen"—when she was three and a half years old. They filed a claim with the court within three years. However, the court would receive a filing from the respondent—a Submission of Evidence Regarding the onset of Autism Spectrum Disorders.

Now the court had to decide on the evidence submitted by the parents of Flora or evidence submitted by HHS. There was no dispute that this child had a form of autism spectrum disorder. The dispute was as to whether the parents had filed a timely petition.

It is the author's opinion that this was the easy and convenient way for the court to dismiss the case instead of determining whether the vaccines did cause a steady decline or promote more aggressive descent into the silent world of autism.

When asked about what can be done to fix or reform a broken system, Gayle was not hesitant to say: (1) Remove the ridiculous three-year filing period, and (2) have Congress change the act to allow parents or individuals whose cases have been dismissed by the court to seek civil remedies. This specific action was made extremely more difficult due to the *Bruesewitz v. Wyeth Labs* court decision by the US Supreme Court in February 2011. The Bruesewitz decision removes the option of exiting out of the program, as Congress originally intended, and forces the petitioner to seek compensation for injuries within the NVICP as an exclusive remedy.

Chapter 6

Statute of Limitations

The statute of limitations as defined in the Vaccine Act is one of the most criticized segments of the act for several reasons. It begins to run "on the date of the occurrence of the first symptom or manifestation of onset or the significant aggravation of such injury."[1] The criticisms of the statute can be defined into two separate dialogues or discussions: 1) the length of time of the statute as compared to other federal and state court systems and jurisdictions; and 2) the interpretation of the actual date of occurrence or onset.

Congress, when establishing the NVICP, was clear on its intentions to provide a quick, efficient, and generous compensation program. What is not clear is the rationale behind the decision to establish limitations of three years for vaccine-related injuries and two years for vaccine-related death. There have been several legislative attempts by Congress to extend the statute from three years to six years, and several recommendations by the ACCV to extend to six or even eight years. However, Congress has defeated every legislative measure to modify the statute, and the HHS Secretary has ignored recommendations from her own advisory committee, the ACCV, to advocate for increasing the length of the statute.

The statute also includes a "look-back" provision for new vaccines or table injuries, which permitted claims for injuries occurring eight years prior to the effective date of revisions to the Vaccine Injury Table, if filed within two years of the statute's effective date.[2] The "look-back" provision would come into play during the addition of the Hepatitis B vaccine to the program in August 1997. This would lead to hundreds of petition filings from individuals claiming vaccine-related injury or death as a result of the administration of the Hepatitis B vaccine after August 6, 1989, and prior to August 6, 1997.[3] The deadline for filing a petition for compensation with the NVICP for injuries resulting from the Hepatitis B vaccine was August 6, 1999.[4] Both human papillomavirus and meningococcal vaccines were added in early 2007 with a look-back period of eight years.

The statute also could be extended by either 1) the discovery rule—extending the time by which a party can file a legal claim until he discovers or should reasonably have discovered the suspected cause of his injury; or 2) the doctrine of equitable tolling—which modifies the statute of limitations in cases of fraud, duress, or similar circumstances.[5]

Congress intended to create a quick and efficient method of adjudication of petitions. Contrary to most federal and state court systems, there is no discovery period allowed by the petitioner. The special master does have the ability to conduct discovery, but only to provide necessary information to render a decision.

Equitable tolling initially was not permitted in the program. Equitable tolling is a legal principal that evolved from the common law of equity.[6] It states that the statute of limitations will not bar a claim if the plaintiff, despite reasonable care and diligent efforts, did not discover the injury until after the limitations period has expired.[7] "Most states toll the statutes of limitations in favor of injured minors," meaning that most state statutes of limitations do not begin to run until the minor reaches the age of majority.[8]

The Vaccine Act is a waiver of the sovereign immunity of the United States because it permits people with a vaccine-related injury, as well as the legal representatives of people who have suffered vaccine-related death, to sue the United States for compensation.[9] The right to sue is not unconditional; the Vaccine Act contains a statute of limitations that places a condition on the waiver of sovereign immunity.[10]

If a vaccine-related injury occurred as a result of the administration of such vaccine, no petition may be filed for compensation under the program for such injury after the expiration of thirty-six months after the date of the occurrence of the first symptom or manifestation of onset or of the significant aggravation of such injury.[11] To put it another way, the United States waives its sovereign immunity only for thirty-six months for vaccine-related injury. After the expiration of the statute, the United States is immune from a lawsuit.

The interpretation of the date of onset of manifestation has been the most criticized element of the ongoing statute of limitations debate. The Vaccine Act requires that a petitioner file documents demonstrating vaccine causation with the petition.[12] Does this suggest that Congress expected petitioners to be able to demonstrate their claims at the time of filing? If so, this is the reason Congress needs to amend the act and extend the statute of limitations by either adding years to the limit or allowing equitable tolling. Congress wrote the legislation with the understanding of the original childhood vaccines and the recommendations from the IOM regarding vaccine-related injuries. At that time, no one anticipated the addition of so many new vaccines in the late 1990s and into the next decade. With these new vaccines, many of the injuries claimed by petitioners were not understood by the medical community. Many of them were autoimmune in nature, many of them affecting the child's behavior or development. Thus, the manifestation of onset of symptoms would not be immediately clear to the medical community or to the parents of these vaccine-injured children. Because of this vague, clouded ability to determine the onset of symptoms, the court would enter into a new era of deciding upon a statute of limitations, which has created a more litigious, more adversarial environment. This is something that Congress did not intend, nor could they have expected this from the NVICP.

There are many petitions that can be highlighted in this chapter regarding the battle of interpreting the date of the onset of symptoms, mostly differences of opinion within the medical community examining the injured child and in determining when the parents noticed a change in behavior or the onset of a medical condition.

Eric

The first petition that I want to share with you is that of Eric and his mother Becky.[13] This case raises questions regarding new vaccines added to the program, with the unknown injuries that can result from the vaccine, and how the medical community identifies the injury and when the first symptom was identified.

Eric's journey with the NVICP begins at his nine-month well-baby checkup. He received the Hepatitis B vaccine and within a few hours developed an acute case of diarrhea. Becky contacted the pediatrician's office and was told by the receptionist that Eric might have picked up a rotavirus during his visit earlier that day. She was told to let nature take its course. Since Becky did not talk with the doctor or a nurse, there was no record of the phone call in Eric's medical chart. And there was no discussion of a possible vaccine reaction.

Later in the evening, Eric developed a fever and started to arch his back and throw his head back. Neither Becky nor her husband had seen or heard about this before. It would be a few years later that she learned from a vaccine expert that Eric's behavior was a clear sign of symptoms of encephalopathy, or brain injury.

Becky would take Eric back to the doctor's office four days later, still battling diarrhea and now fevers. The pediatrician examined Eric and told her that Eric showed no signs of distress and that he was properly hydrated. Over the course of the next two years, there would be a total of twenty-one visits or phone calls to the doctor. Becky started to notice a decline in the overall health of her son.

It was two years from Eric's first big reaction to the Hepatitis B vaccine that he also received a diagnosis of autism, in the fall of 2000. Becky was also introduced to other parents in Southern California who had witnessed autism in their own children.

Then the research started—what to do with her son, how to help him. The journey to recovery for Eric started in January of 2001. Becky found a local doctor who specialized in the DAN! protocol (Defeat Autism Now). The doctor assisted Becky in obtaining the necessary lab work in order to help Eric overcome his vitamin and mineral deficiencies.

In the spring of 2002, Becky was contacted by a local attorney who filed a civil tort lawsuit in November of that same year. The attorney learned later that the case could not go forward and that all vaccine-related-injury claims had to be filed in the NVICP.

Eric's vaccine injury claim was then turned over to an attorney from Portland, Oregon, who filed a petition with the NVICP in November of 2004. His petition was placed into the large omnibus that was forming to handle all the autism claims. This omnibus was called the Omnibus Autism Proceeding (OAP) and would eventually contain over 5,500 petitions.

In the fall of 2007, Eric's petition had been selected as a possible test case for the second round of cases to be heard starting in May 2008. The second-round test cases comprised petitions that claimed that a mercury-based preservative, thimerosal, was the cause of the vaccine injury. The first round of test cases comprised petitions that claimed the MMR-plus-thimerosal-containing vaccines caused a vaccine injury.

Then the bottom fell out. The lead attorneys representing all of the petitions filed in the OAP contacted Becky and told her that the petition was time-barred. The respondent, represented by DOJ attorneys, found a handwritten note, inscribed on the side of one of Eric's medical charts, stating the pediatrician on the twenty-month well-baby checkup, wrote "mild speech delay." This note was not conveyed to the parents; they had no idea or any conversation with the pediatrician about the doctor's concern during that visit. To Becky, the petition was filed within the three-year statute of limitations. Eric was formally diagnosed with autism in November of 2000. The family filed a vaccine-injury claim in November of 2002.[14] The program accepted the original civil filing date of November 2002.

Becky's attorney told her that the DOJ starts the clock at the first medically documented symptom of injury. Unbeknownst to Becky, Eric's pediatrician wrote a note to herself at his twenty-month checkup that said "mild speech delay." The checkup was September 14, 1999. This puts the time limit at three years, six weeks. Because of this determination, the petition would be withdrawn from consideration as a test case and placed back into the OAP with the other 5,500 petitions.

The petition was dismissed in February 2012.[15]

Markovich v. HHS

The defining case or precedential case for interpreting when the statute starts to run under the Vaccine Act is *Markovich v. HHS*. The government's position was that the limitations period begins with the first sign or symptom or manifestation of onset of a condition, regardless of whether it is recognized as a sign or symptom of an injury at the time.[16] Petitioner argued that the first sign or symptom or manifestation of onset means something that is manifest, i.e., something that is understood to be a sign or symptom of a vaccine injury.[17]

In order to understand the arguments from both the petitioner and the respondent, let's wind the clock back to July 10, 2000, when the little girl received several vaccinations during her two-month well-baby checkup. At this visit, she received DTaP, IPV, and HiB vaccinations.[18]

According to medical records, she had some rapid eye blinking later that day as witnessed by her parents. In an affidavit filed with the court, the mother "thought she was just sleepy, but now I am aware she may have been having seizures between the time of the immunization and August 30, 2000, when she had her first serious episode that required hospitalization."[19] This would be the critical fulcrum that tilted the hands of justice toward the respondent in the eyes of the special master.

The respondent contends "that because the little girl's rapid eye blinking of July 10, 2000, was the first symptom of her seizure disorder, the plain language of the statute requires that the 36-month period began running on that date. The limitation's period is triggered by the first symptom or manifestation of onset, not by the Petitioner's actual knowledge or awareness of a claim arising under the Vaccine Act. The Petitioners need not know that their child suffered a vaccine-related injury. Rather, it is sufficient that these parents were aware of the July 10, 2000, eye-blinking episode; the parents need not have been aware of the significance."[20]

The parents of this little girl, also having to deal with the constant seizures and other medical conditions, filed a petition with the NVICP on August 29, 2003. The special master dismissed the petition due to a lack of jurisdiction, and the statute of limitations had expired six weeks earlier.

In what is considered well-settled law, the Vaccine Act does not require a diagnosis of a condition to start the running of the statute of limitations.[21] Also, the Vaccine Act does not require knowledge that the vaccine caused the symptom or manifestation of onset in order for the statute of limitations to start running.[22]

So where does that leave us? The little girl noted above still requires medical care for her seizures and speech delay. The case had the potential to award a large compensable damage award to provide the funding for the constant medical care this child requires on a daily basis.

In the similar matter, the little boy Eric has grown to be a young teen who still needs the constant attention of his parents. He is learning to manage and live with his autism, and is possibly one of the test cases that actually received a hearing instead of being dismissed.

Medical professionals need to make sure that parents are aware of all notes and medical records in order to prevent what happened to Eric and his parents. Parents and their doctors need to have open and honest discussions of what can happen after administration of any vaccination. Otherwise, we will head toward a more adversarial and hostile environment, as shown in the following statements regarding *Pertnoy v. HHS*.

The need to expand the current statute of limitations can be demonstrated by the following special master's rationalization of her decision to deny compensation by reasoning that "under an objective standard a reasonable parent would have inquired into her legal rights . . . after seeing such drastic changes in her son's condition."[23] In that case, the child's "parents made a good faith effort and exercised due diligence in attempting to discover the causes of the boy's injuries. Why would his parents have thought to pursue legal remedies if they did not even have evidence to prove a causal relationship between his injuries and the vaccination?"[24] If every parent performed their duty, as stated by Special Master Laura Millman, only absurd results would come, since parents would be encouraged to call their attorneys and think about litigation during a time when they are focusing on trying to make their children healthier.[25]

Extending the statute of limitations, while perhaps subjecting the government to more liability, would go a long way toward easing the fears of potential petitioners who would otherwise be unable to obtain sufficient information to lodge a complete complaint.[26]

I will offer and discuss in a later chapter the idea that if Congress decides to expand the statute of limitations, they should also instruct the court to allow all the petitions that were dismissed on this technicality to re-apply for compensation of a vaccine-related injury or death.

Michelle Staley

Here is another heartbreaking story, this one of a health-care worker who in 1994 and 1995 received the Hepatitis B vaccination. The Hepatitis B vaccine was not adopted into the program until 1997. Therefore, Michelle was one of several thousand who could file a petition with the program as a "pre-act" case. The deadline for filing a petition with the program was August 6, 1999. The other issue here is the complete failure of the HHS Secretary to conduct public awareness campaigns for the program as mandated by Congress.

Following her first set of vaccinations in 1994, Michelle was extremely tired. She sought medical care for her constant fatigue. Her next vaccination of Hepatitis B was in 1995. After receiving that vaccine, she was extremely tired, could not work as a health-care practitioner, and could not stand on her feet for more than a couple of minutes at a time. In August of 1995, she visited a doctor who diagnosed her with chronic fatigue syndrome.

But she would not improve and continued to seek out medical doctors who could help her with her constant fatigue. It was August 2003, nearly eight years later, when a doctor diagnosed her with Chronic Autoimmune Encephalomyelitis caused by the Hepatitis B vaccine.[27] This was the first time that Michelle would be told that her medical condition was caused by a vaccine.

For the previous nine years, since her first Hepatitis B vaccination, she had been struggling to find the source of her chronic fatigue. None of the medical doctors whom she had seen as a patient made any connection. So she started to research what, if any, options she had to protect her interests. She filed for social security disability benefits. And she attempted to file a petition with the NVICP. She sought the legal assistance, according to records filed with the NVICP, of nearly thirty different attorneys, some of whom did not practice in the program. All of them turned her down due to their analysis of the statute of limitations.

Michelle would finally file a petition with the program in August of 2006, twelve years after receiving her first Hepatitis B vaccination.

The respondent filed a motion with the court to dismiss the petition due to exceeding the statute of limitations. The special master conducted a status conference with Michelle and the DOJ attorney representing the respondent. The special master agreed with the respondent's motion to dismiss on the grounds that the petition is time-barred.

This is another clear case of a petitioner not being aware of the program, many doctors in denial of vaccine-related injury, and the HHS Secretary refusing to inform the public about the program as mandated by Congress and clearly outlined in statute. The Supreme Court explains the purpose and origin of statutes of limitations thusly:

> Statutes of limitation find their justification in necessity and convenience rather than in logic. They represent expedients, rather than principles. They are practical and pragmatic devices to spare the courts from litigation of stale claims, and a citizen from being put to his defense after memories have faded, witnesses have died or disappeared, and evidence has been lost. They are by definition arbitrary, and their operation does not discriminate between the just and the unjust claim, or the voidable and unavoidable delay.[28]

If only this were the case. It appears that Congress and the Supreme Court have it wrong when it comes to the program and the hundreds of vaccine-injured petitioners who cannot present their petition and be heard on the merits of the case. It is definitely not about memories faded, or witnesses who disappeared; it is about the justice that has died for so many.

Chapter 7

Redaction Rule 18(b)

One of the most contentious issues within the NVICP is the topic of redaction. This is the ability to remove certain personal information from a decision, opinion, or order to protect personal medical history and the identity of the injured party. And in my opinion, even the most generous decision in favor of the petitioner has not gone far enough to protect personal information from being invaded by those individuals and organizations that use this information to intimidate petitioners and thus discourage the filing of many petitions for vaccine injury.

Special masters derive their powers from the Vaccine Act of 1986 and subsequent amendments by Congress in 1989.[1] Vaccine Rule 18(b) allows a special master or a judge to redact certain information from any decision, opinion, or order.[2] A decision of the special master or judge in the Federal Court of Claims will be held for fourteen days to allow each party an opportunity to object to a public disclosure of any information furnished by that party. A redaction motion must be filed within the fourteen-day period. The motion also must include a proposed redacted version of the decision. The criteria for redacting are as follows:[3]

> One, a trade secret or commercial or financial in substance and is privileged or confidential; or
> Two, includes medical files or other documents of a similar nature, the disclosure of which would constitute a clear unwarranted invasion of privacy.

Any objecting party must provide the court with the proposed redacted version of the decision; in the absence of any objection the entire decision will be made public.[4] Rule 18(b) provides no specific guidance concerning the type of disclosure of medical files or similar files that "constitute a clearly unwarranted invasion of privacy."[5] This could be interpreted as providing the special masters with discretion on interpretation of the rule.

In 1986 when Congress passed the National Childhood Vaccine Injury Act (NCVIA) establishing a specialized court and proceedings for persons who have been injured by vaccines or those family members who died as a result of a vaccine, the act also was intended to advance the public health through the collection and dissemination of information about vaccines, including adverse events potentially related to vaccine administration, and through promoting the development of safer vaccines.[6]

The entire federal court system is governed by the E-Government Act of 2002 regarding disclosure of personal information and privacy, which instructed the judiciary to make its records electronically accessible to the public. The E-Government Act affirms that the public has an interest in obtaining access to court filings and decisions, but recognizes that some information is private, sensitive, and should not be publicly disclosed.

Section 205 of the E-Government Act provides that all federal courts shall establish and maintain a website that provides public access to court rules, docket information, and the substance of all written opinions, among other information.[7] As this relates to the Vaccine Act, decisions and orders are published on the website of the court of Federal Claims.

The Vaccine Act of 1986 limits the authority to redact decisions. The Vaccine Act permits redaction upon request for medical information that, if disclosed, would constitute a "clearly unwarranted invasion of privacy." Neither the statute nor the legislative history provides explicit guidance as to the content of the quoted phrase.

In order to understand where personal information may be disclosed, there are four areas of disclosure:[8]

First, Congress mandated that the HHS Secretary publish a list of all vaccine claims in the Federal Register.[9] The express purpose of this provision was to disseminate information concerning vaccine injury claims, to foster public awareness and to permit public comment.

Second, Congress protected information submitted by claimants in the course of adjudication. Thus, treatment records and similar documentation containing personal medical records are closed to the public view. The purpose of this provision is to protect personal or medical and other information, the public disclosure of which is deemed by Congress to be unnecessary to carrying out the statutory purposes.

Third, Congress required publication of special masters' decisions. This is consistent with the traditional presumption of affording public access to judicial actions and serves the Vaccine Act's express purpose in promoting public awareness of vaccine safety.

Fourth, Congress conferred authority on special masters to redact a narrow subset of personal information, including certain medical information, upon a specific showing satisfying the criteria for redaction set forth in subsections 12(d)4(b) i & ii of the Vaccine Act.

A special master is not authorized to alter the balance between public and private interests that Congress put in the Vaccine Act; special masters' authority is limited to that granted by Congress.[10] Under the plain provisions of the Vaccine Act, and consistent with the statutory scheme, a special master's discretion to order redaction is therefore limited. It does not extend beyond redacting information as described in section 12(d)4(b).[11]

In recent months petitioners and their attorneys have been struggling when asking the court to redact personal medical history, names, addresses, local clinics, doctors, and other information that links the decision to the specific petitioner. The fourteen-day rule to file a motion to redact has been met with great resistance from the court, especially when filing a motion to redact an order or decision while the petition is still being heard.

Recently there was an incident regarding a special master's decision on publishing a Findings of Fact decision regarding a petition that is still pending in the NVICP. The mother representing her deceased daughter has been a strong advocate, speaking out in the public regarding vaccine safety. She recently appeared on a nationally televised talk show to discuss what she and her attorney claim—the death of her daughter was caused by a specific vaccine. The published decision clearly presented a detailed look at medical history testimony and other medical records, and it was preliminary. More hearings and testimony would follow. To go by this decision would only lead to an incomplete analysis of the incomplete record. This information was posted on the court's website; names and other personal information were included and should've been redacted, but were not.

This decision was obtained by an Internet blogger who clearly used the information to publicly embarrass and intimidate the mother in an attempt to discredit her fight and her opinions of what happened to her daughter. This blogger had no vested interests in this decision other than to purposely and maliciously attack the mother. This is not what Congress intended to have happen. This blogger has a history of not advancing public discourse and discussion about vaccine safety, but rather using a blog to intimidate and embarrass those who do not share his narrow viewpoint of vaccines and vaccine injury.

Judge Lettow, of the Federal Court of Claims, in his opinion and order in the matter of *W. C. v. HHS*, wrote that "these purposes are not served by requiring petitioners' names to be published even where an objection is made on reasonable grounds. Such disclosures may discourage potential petitioners from filing new cases, thus tending to inhibit public awareness of vaccines and their risks. Importantly, in this vein, the Senate Committee Report on the bill that became the Vaccine Act of 1986 specified that the committee did not believe that the name of the individual who suffered an adverse reaction need be made available to the public."

In light of the different public purposes behind disclosure in civil and vaccine cases, and the strength of the connection between the terms of the Freedom of Information Act (FOIA) and those of the Vaccine Act, the special master erred in relying on precedents from the 9th Circuit regarding criteria for the designation of anonymous plaintiffs as a basis for interpretation of the privacy provisions of the Vaccine Act.

In another decision on redaction, *C. S. v. HHS*, the special master granted redaction of the individual's name and ordered all decisions to insert the initials of the petitioner. In his motion to redact, the petitioner had claimed that "disclosure of his name linked to his medical conditions will result in a clearly unwarranted invasion of his privacy interest."[12] The petitioner had asked for his name to be removed and his initials inserted due to privacy concerns that the case would jeopardize his career and effectiveness in the classroom with his students and the students' parents.[13] This redaction did not totally eliminate the petitioner's name from the public view—it is just a partial redaction.

In another redaction decision, *A. K. v. HHS*, the special master was asked to rule on a motion from the petitioner to remove her name and medical condition from all decisions. The respondent (the HHS Secretary) objected to the motion, stating the petitioner had failed to provide a sufficient basis for redaction of information regarding her medical condition.[14] The special master granted the petitioner's motion in part and denied it in part.[15] The petitioner was able to remove her name from the petition and replace it with her initials. However, her request to remove her medical condition was denied.

It is extremely important that petitioners who are requesting the redaction of personal information file motions within fourteen days of the judgment date of any decision or order. The following case discussion is about a mother of three children, all of them filing petitions with the NVICP claiming vaccine injuries. All three petitions were dismissed and compensation was denied. During the application for attorney fees and costs, which have separate filing date requirements (180 days from judgment), redaction motions were included asking to redact all three children's names from the final judgment decisions. The special master denied all three redaction motions. The motions were filed in a timely manner, but because there were no redaction motions filed for the entitlement decisions, granting the relief requested at this time would not protect the petitioners' privacy, as they had been named in the published entitlement decision.[16]

However, the redaction process is not consistent even when decided by the same special master. A petitioner was granted full redaction due to his career as a member of the DEA. He argued that knowledge of his compensation award would jeopardize his ability to continue his work as an undercover officer. Yet another petitioner who was awarded compensation from the same special master was denied redaction. In her motion, the petitioner argued that her husband worked as an undercover police officer and that she was also estranged from her father, resulting from having received compensation. The petitioner asked to have her name removed, initials inserted, and any references to her husband or her work history completely removed.

Thus we ask Congress to reexamine the statute regarding redaction to prevent future episodes of unwanted and unnecessary disclosure of personal information that has no relevance to the study of vaccine safety.

Chapter 8

Proving Off-Table Injuries

As I briefly covered earlier, the NCVIA (the act itself) was void of guidance on how the court was to deal with off-table injuries; debate or discussion on the matter was negligible, according to the Congressional record. The court, struggling with how to create standards for adjudicating petitions, created inconsistent methods. Often, this led to some punitive decisions, thus creating another problem.

Congress' intent for the Vaccine Act was to have a less adversarial case adjudication than typical tort claims.[1] Petitioners needed only to prove they suffered a vaccine injury; no one inquired into whether the manufacturer or any other party was negligent.[2]

Many petitions would turn into litigious events, with motions for review filed with the Federal Court of Claims and appeals filed with the Federal Circuit Court of Appeals. Because of this litigious environment facing petitioners who filed claims of off-table injury or death, the length of time before a complete adjudication of their case, for many of these petitioners, would easily top five to ten years, if not longer. This was hardly the intent of Congress, which had wanted to provide a quick and efficient method to determine compensation of vaccine-related injuries and death.

In one of the earliest Federal Circuit decisions (July 1991) on causal proof in off-table cases, *Hines v. Secretary of Health & Human Services*, the court defined the issue before the special master as "whether the evidence submitted by the Petitioner warranted a conclusion that the vaccine caused the injury."[3] Relying on the arbitrary and capricious standard of review,[4] the *Hines* court made clear that just what type of evidence and how much of it a petitioner had to present to merit such a conclusion generally was left to the special master's discretion.[5]

On the heels of the *Hines* decision came another case that led the court to develop an even more stringent and concise baseline to develop decisions. In *Grant v. Secretary of Health and Human Services,* in February 1992, the Federal Court of Claims drafted a specific, three-part test to prove causation in fact: Petitioners had to 1) "show a medical theory causally connecting the vaccination and the injury"; 2) offer "proof of a logical sequence of cause and effect showing that the vaccination was the reason for the injury"; and 3) support the "logical sequence of cause and effect" with a "reputable medical or scientific explanation."[6] Once the petitioner satisfied these criteria, the special master had to evaluate whether, based on a preponderance of the evidence, factors not related to the vaccine could have caused the injury.[7] The court in the *Grant* decision established that to receive award of compensation two findings were required to be determined by the special master: causation-in-fact and the absence of an alternative cause of injury.[8] Although the burden clearly fell on the petitioner to establish causation-in-fact, the courts struggled with whether the petitioner or the respondent bore the burden of proving the absence of an alternative etiology.[9]

Later cases relied heavily upon the *Grant* framework for causal proof requirements. These cases, borrowing from the general causation factor in toxic tort cases, viewed the first factor, demonstrating a medical theory linking the vaccine to the injury, as requiring the petitioner to establish that the vaccine can in theory cause the injury suffered. The second factor, showing a "logical sequence of cause and effect" between the vaccine and the injury by applying the proffered medical theory, bridged the connection from the theoretical to the injury in the claim at hand, and was similar to the specific causation factor of toxic tort cases. To satisfy this second factor, petitioners often had to demonstrate a temporal link between the vaccine and the injury and eliminate alternative causes of the injury. Merely meeting one or both of these criteria was not enough to establish a preponderance of the evidence, however. The third factor, "reputable" medical or scientific support, indicated that a petitioner must provide reliable evidence to support the second factor, but the test for reliability was not clearly defined.

Under these cases, appellate review emphasized the broad discretion granted to the special masters, and the outcome of off-table claims depended almost entirely on the special masters' acceptance and interpretation of weighing the evidence with regard to causation. On review, the Federal Circuit examined three factors: whether the special master 1) "considered the relevant evidence of record"; 2) had "drawn plausible inferences"; and 3) "articulated a rational basis for the decision." If the special master performed all three tasks, reversible error would be "extremely difficult to demonstrate." Given the broad discretion and high degree of appellate deference afforded the special masters, it is difficult to determine consistent patterns of evidence standards in early Federal Circuit off-table cases.

Some consistencies did surface, however. The best evidence, pathological markers, was considered virtually dispositive from the start, but most vaccines simply leave no such footprints. Similarly, these early cases gave great weight to epidemiological studies demonstrating a relative risk greater than 2.0, similar to the toxic tort arena. Given the limited availability of these two forms of evidence, however, petitioners turned to weaker, circumstantial evidence to prove causation, such as animal studies, case reports, treating physician's testimony, medical textbooks, and comparable biological mechanisms. Special masters struggled with how to evaluate such evidence, and, in employing the Grant test, the special masters applied inconsistent standards to the same kinds of evidence and reached inconsistent results. They also struggled with what combinations of evidence sufficiently demonstrated causation.

Another issue on which the vaccine courts did not agree was whether the petitioner had to proffer a precise biological or immunological mechanism that explained how the injury arose from the vaccine. The Federal Circuit's response to the special masters' confusion did nothing to alleviate it. Instead, the Federal Circuit emphasized their discretion by stressing the importance of looking at the totality of evidence in determining causation. In *Jay v. Secretary of Health & Human Services*, for example, the Federal Circuit reversed a grant of summary judgment to the government, remanding the case for an award of compensation (July 1993). The petitioners alleged that a DPT vaccination caused encephalopathy, which in turn led to their son's death. The special master held that the medical expert could not establish encephalopathy based only on the prolonged crying that followed the vaccine, but the Federal Circuit ruled that the special master had failed to consider the evidence as a whole, particularly the temporal association and the fact that a death occurred. It held that the petitioners were entitled to compensation:

> The undisputed facts of record . . . include that an otherwise healthy child received a DPT shot; the DPT shot caused fever, directly or indirectly limpness, and intermittent inconsolable extended screaming; the child missed his normal nightly feeding; the child died within 18 hours of the shot; the autopsy was inconclusive; and a medical expert testified, un-

contradicted, that the DPT shot caused the death, the medical theory being that an encephalopathy occurred. . . . We therefore hold as a matter of law that on the undisputed facts of record a reasonable person could not conclude that the Jays failed to prove that the DPT vaccine was the likely cause of Matthew's death.[10]

Because the government did not dispute any of the petitioners' evidence, the medical records, the autopsy report, the parents' testimony, and medical expert testimony were sufficient to prove causation-in-fact. The Federal Circuit thus indicated that the floor for sufficiency on an off-table claim was low and highly contextual, and the government's lack of evidence could support the petitioner's claim in favor of finding causation. The Federal Circuit also resisted efforts to apply *Daubert* to test expert testimony. For example, in *Golub v. Secretary of Health & Human Services*, the petitioner alleged that a DPT vaccination caused meningitis, which in turn caused a seizure disorder, developmental delay, and cortical damage. The special master denied compensation because the petitioner's theory, although plausible, did not "rise to the level of scientific reliability."[11] The special master dismissed evidence of a temporal relationship, animal studies, and studies involving HIV patients, and dismissed a study involving children because it was not peer-reviewed or published.[12] Eschewing application of *Daubert* standards to this context, the Federal Circuit countered that a petitioner's expert theory on causation only had to be "reasonably reliable" and did not need to "rise to the level of being a scientific certainty."[13] The court clarified that "while a proximate temporal association alone does not establish a causal link between the vaccination and the injury, where a strong temporal relationship exists, the additional showing of a reasonable medical theory causally connecting the vaccination and the injury would suffice to establish a causal link."[14]

Finally, the Federal Circuit relied on the confusing substantial factor test from the *Second Restatement of Torts* when more than one suspected causal factor existed.[15] In *Shyface v. Secretary of Health & Human Services*, for example, the petitioner's expert testified that the combination of the DPT vaccine and an unrelated factor—E. coli pneumonia—caused death. The expert testified that the death would not have occurred had only one of the factors been present and that it could not be determined which factor contributed more to the death. The government's expert disagreed, testifying that the E. coli infection alone caused the death. The special master denied compensation because the petitioners could not prove that the vaccine caused the death, and the court of Federal Claims upheld the denial, requiring the petitioners to establish the vaccine as the "predominant cause" of death in order to prevail. On appeal, the petitioners argued for a broader causal test requiring them to establish only that the vaccine was a "but-for," not the "predominant," cause of death. The Federal Circuit stated that "the Vaccine Act's requirement of causation in non-table cases was not viewed as distinct from causation in the tort law" and "adopted the *Second Restatement rule* for purposes of determining vaccine injury, that an action was the 'legal cause' of harm if that action is a 'substantial factor' in bringing about the harm, and that the harm would not have occurred but for the action."[16] Because, in the Federal Circuit's estimation, the "undisputed" facts established that the DPT vaccine was both a substantial factor and a *but-for* cause of the death, the court held that the petitioners were entitled to compensation.[17]

Thus, the Federal Circuit's jurisprudence gave minimal guidance to the special masters on the type and amount of causal proof to demand of petitioners and ignored the developments occurring in the tort context for causal proof. This lack of guidance resulted in disarray in the program.

Althen—Current Standard for Proving Causation of Off-Table Injury

The court continued to struggle developing a consistent framework for decisions regarding claims of off-table injuries. As the court evolved from *Hines* to *Grant* to *Stevens*, the Federal Circuit Court of Appeals finally arrived at a standard that was consistent, fair, and equitable for all parties with *Althen v. HHS* (2005). Basically, it gave the petitioner a fighting chance. Prior to *Althen*, the standard developed under *Stevens v. HHS* (1999) swung the pendulum too far in favor of the respondent. The burden of proof was extremely high and was not in accordance with the wishes of Congress. As one attorney who represents many petitioners told me, "it was too damn punitive."

The Federal Circuit Court of Appeals, in their deliberations for *Althen v. HHS*, noted that the act provides for an establishment of causation in one of two ways: through a statutorily prescribed presumption of causation by showing that an injury falls within the vaccine injury table; or, when the complained of injury is not listed in the vaccine injury table, by proving causation in fact. In any case, the petitioner must prove by a preponderance of the evidence that the vaccine caused the injury.[18]

To meet the preponderance standard, the petitioner must show a medical theory causally connecting the vaccination and the injury.[19] A persuasive medical theory is demonstrated by proof of a logical sequence of cause and effect showing that the vaccination was the reason for the injury, the logical sequence being supported by reputable medical or scientific explanation, i.e., evidence in the form of scientific studies or expert medical testimony.[20]

The petitioner may recover compensation if they show that the vaccine was not only a *but-for* cause of the injury but also a substantial factor in bringing about the injury.[21] The petitioner's burden is to show by a preponderance of evidence that the vaccination brought about the injury by providing: 1) a medical theory causally connecting the vaccination and the injury; 2) a logical sequence of cause and effect showing that the vaccination was a reason for the injury; and 3) a showing of the proximate temporal relationship between vaccination and injury. If the petitioner satisfies this burden, then the petitioner is entitled to recover compensation unless the government shows, also by a preponderance of evidence, that the injury was in fact caused by factors unrelated to the vaccine.[22]

In *Althen*, the Federal Circuit quoted its opinion:[23]

> A persuasive medical theory is demonstrated by "proof of a logical sequence of cause and effect showing that the vaccination was the reason for the injury," the logical sequence being supported by "reputable medical or scientific explanation," i.e., "evidence in the form of scientific studies or expert medical testimony." Without more, "evidence showing an absence of other causes does not meet Petitioners' affirmative duty to show actual or legal causation." Mere temporal association is not sufficient to prove causation in fact.

With *Althen*, the petitioner had a more equitable opportunity to proceed with their claim. As with many other aspects of the program, the entire process is more about policy than adjudicating claims of the petitioners based upon a preponderance of evidence. After *Althen*, there would be considerable pressure to chisel away at the standards by special masters and judges and their word-smithing decisions and interpretations.

Decisions Regarding Significant Aggravation Claims

The Vaccine Act defined significant aggravation as "any change for the worse in a preexisting condition which results in a markedly greater disability, pain, or illness accompanied by substantial deterioration of health."[24] Congress stated that petitioners who bring significant aggravation claims cannot receive compensation for conditions that might legitimately be described as preexisting (e.g., a child with monthly seizures who, after vaccination, has seizures every three and a half weeks), but is meant to encompass serious deterioration (e.g., a child with monthly seizures who, after vaccination, has seizures on a daily basis).[25]

Special masters consistently struggled with their decisions regarding significant aggravation even though the Vaccine Act specifies that significant aggravation and new injury circumstances constitute separate avenues to potential recovery or damages.[26]

In 1991, *Misasi v. HHS* allowed the court for the first time to create a legal construct for handling significant aggravation cases. Under the Misasi framework, to evaluate whether a person has suffered a significant aggravation of a preexisting condition, the special master must 1) assess the individual's condition prior to administration of the vaccine, i.e., evaluate the nature and extent of the individual's preexisting condition; 2) assess the individual's current condition after administration of the vaccine; 3) predict the individual's condition had the vaccine not been administered; and 4) compare the individual's current condition with the predicted condition had the vaccine not been administered. Only if the person's current condition is significantly worse than the person's predicted condition had the vaccine not been administered is the petitioner entitled to compensation.[27]

The inconsistent decisions continued until the Federal Circuit Court of Appeals, in their remand decision of *Whitecotton v. HHS*, articulated a four-part test to govern significant aggravation for on-table claims. The Whitecotton test required the special master to:[28]

1. assess the person's condition prior to administration of the vaccine;
2. assess the person's current condition; and

3. determine if the person's current condition constitutes a significant aggravation of the person's condition prior to the vaccination within the meaning of the statute. If the special master concludes that the person has suffered significant aggravation, they must then

4. determine whether the symptom or the manifestation of the significant aggravation occurred within the time period prescribed by the vaccine injury table.

So now we have a binding decision by the Federal Circuit Court of Appeals that instructs the special masters and the Federal Court of Claims on how to govern significant aggravation claims for on-table injuries.

A more complex, detailed decision was upcoming regarding how to handle significant aggravation claims for off-table injuries. The Federal Circuit Court of Appeals, in *Loving v. HHS*, created a framework combining the Althen test standard with their decision in *Whitecotton v. HHS*. The new Loving standard said that a preponderance of evidence existed if the petitioner could show the following:

1. the person's condition prior to administration of the vaccine;

2. the person's current condition or the condition following the vaccination if that is also pertinent;

3. whether the person's current condition constitutes a significant aggravation of the person's condition prior to vaccination;

4. a medical theory causally connecting such a significant worsened condition to the vaccination;

5. a logical sequence of cause and effect showing that the vaccination was the reason for the significant aggravation; and

6. a showing of an approximate temporal relationship between the vaccination and the significant aggravation.

If the petitioner is able to successfully put forward such a *prima facie* case, the burden shifts to the respondent to prove by a preponderance of evidence that the petitioner's significant aggravation was caused by some factor other than the vaccine.[29] With significant aggravation claims, "once a Petitioner has made a prima facie case, the government may still prevail if it can show, to a preponderance of evidence, that the pre-existing condition was, in fact, the cause of an individual's post-vaccination significant aggravation."[30] In addition, the government may be able to point to other factors apart from the pre-existing condition that demonstrate the vaccine did not cause a significant aggravation.[31]

The current process of adjudicating petitions in the NVICP has turned into an adversarial, full litigation instead of the no-fault, quick, generous program that Congress designed. In the early years of the program, most petitions, nearly 90 percent of them, were adjudicated as on-table injuries, thus the time from filing to the completion of the process was under two years' time. Today, we are at the opposite end of the spectrum. Most claims, estimated at up to 90 percent of petitions that are not dismissed because of being time-barred or because of lack of jurisdiction, are now off-table claims, requiring medical expert testimony; these claims have become litigious and adversarial, something that Congress did not want to happen.

Chapter 9

Death

To lose a child to cancer or because of an automobile accident is traumatic for every family. It is devastating. We are not supposed to outlive our children. So how do we as parents deal with the loss of our child due to the rare event of death by vaccination?

We have been programmed by media and our medical community that vaccination is for the greater good. It is done to protect the herd and public health. It is accepted that there might be a rare incident of injury or worse. This is why there is a National Vaccine Injury Compensation Program. But the other part of that equation—the casualties of the so-called greater good—is not just a statistic on paper.

The victims are our flesh and blood. They are our family members, our brothers and sisters, our mothers and fathers, cousins, nieces, and nephews. Most families today can look over their entire family and acknowledge someone who is struggling with a disability. Many families now acknowledge someone within their family who was injured by a vaccine. The figure is not as small as the medical community and our own government wants us to believe. And there is a growing subset of families dealing with the loss of a family member due to some form of a vaccine. The incidents of death by vaccine are not as rare as we are led to believe.

In our society, we value life with extreme high regard. Why is it that we do not value the loss of life by vaccine injury the same way? In courtrooms across the nation, decisions are being made, juries awarding damages, or settlements being agreed, awarding compensable monetary damages ranging from hundreds of thousands of dollars to several million dollars for the accidental loss of life.

The Vaccine Act provides that the estate of a deceased person may recover up to $250,000 when a vaccine causes a person's death.[1] Some families who have won compensation might only receive $30,000 or $75,000 as part of a stipulation or agreement; some do receive the cap limit of $250,000. What is yet to be determined, however, is whether an estate can recover additional compensation for pain and suffering, emotional distress, lost earnings, and medical expenses. It was only within the last few years that the program started to award pain-and-suffering damages up to $250,000. Yet there are many families who have been turned away, mainly due to not being able to locate a medical expert who will testify about why the newborn child died four days after the Hepatitis B vaccine was administered, or why the senior citizen died from complications of GBS as a result of an influenza vaccine administered four months earlier.

The government typically denies that the vaccine contributed to the death, pointing to reports from the medical examiner showing the cause of death as SIDS or "cause unknown." Members of the medical profession who step forward to support families who believe that their loved one died from vaccine injury often receive harsh treatment from the Department of Justice. There are several examples of the government attacking the petitioner's expert witnesses.

The heart and spirit of the NVICP as established in 1988 was to provide a "no-fault" means of adjudicating petitions in a fair, quick, generous, and compassionate manner. Nothing is quick when most death petitions filed since the beginning take an average of five to seven years, with several taking a decade or longer, to determine whether damages are to be awarded.

Nothing is fair or compassionate when a family cannot hire a medical expert due to the high cost, a medical expert who could testify that the vaccine the child received two days earlier contributed to the death of that child. Nothing is generous when the original statute provided for "up to" $250,000 with an inflation index to be included for future awards. The inflation index was removed the following year in one of Congress' reconciliation budget bills. It's highly unlikely that the inflation index was going to break the bank, so who actually removed the index from the statute? No one really knows, just like many other times in Congress when legislation is modified or altered, or an amendment is included in the middle of the night.

Congress needs to address this compensation award by bringing it up to the levels at which other federal and state courts have consistently awarded damages. There have been proposals to increase the benefit level up to $500,000 or even to $1,000,000. But for most families, the compensation doesn't reflect the damage caused by the loss of a child or loved one.

To help you better understand how the court has decided the death benefit in specific cases, let me first review the evolution of the statute and how it is applied to today's petitions. While the original statute allowed a compensation amount of up to $250,000, the court has debated and often ruled against certain cases in regards to additional damages beyond the death benefit.

One such case is 1994's *Zatuchni v. HHS*. In *Zatuchni*, Ms. Snyder, the original petitioner, filed a claim seeking compensation for an off-table injury caused by a Rubella vaccination. Her petition remained pending for several years. In April 2005 Ms. Snyder died, and eight days later the special master ruled against her injury claim. Ms. Zatuchni, Executrix of the Estate of E. Barbara Snyder, filed a motion with the court to become the representative of the Snyder estate.

Upon review in the United States Court of Federal Claims, Judge Wheeler reversed the decision, "stating that the special master set the burden of proof bar too high for the petitioner and not high enough for the respondent, in light of the Federal Circuit Court of Appeals' decision in *Althen*, several months prior."

The court remanded the case back to the original special master to determine if Ms. Snyder's death was due to the vaccine, therefore entitling the estate to the death benefit. On remand, the special master determined that Ms. Snyder's death was indeed the result of the vaccine, and awarded the estate the death benefit without additional compensation.

The petitioner filed a motion for review with the court of Federal Claims claiming that the special master's decision awarding only a death benefit is contrary to law, claiming that a simple reading of the Vaccine Act should permit the recovery of a death benefit and any economic losses caused by the vaccine. The Court heard oral arguments on August 17, 2006, and determined that the special master's decision on remand is not in accordance with law. The court would not accept the argument from the respondent that an injured party who suffered thirteen years of economic losses during her lifetime somehow forfeited those losses by dying while her case was pending before the court. On October 16, 2006, the court vacated the special master's decision on remand and adopted the special master's findings from the original decision regarding economic losses.

The respondent appealed this decision to the Federal Circuit Court of Appeals. On February 12, 2008, in a split decision 2–1 that took fourteen years from when the petition was filed, the Federal Circuit Court of Appeals affirmed the decision of the Federal Court of Claims.

The Federal Circuit ruled in favor of Ms. Zatuchni as administrator of Ms. Snyder's estate and rejected the respondent's argument by stating "the fact that a vaccine-related death followed a vaccine-related injury in a particular case does not alter the fact that certain expenses were incurred, wages lost, or pain-and-suffering endured in the interim, and these damages are no less related to or caused by a vaccine-related injury within the meaning of subsections(a)(1), (3), and (4) simply because the vaccine-injured person in question is no longer living; thus, it is in no way inconsistent with the text of the statute to award compensation under the above subsections for damages that resulted from or were sustained by reason of a vaccine-related injury in addition to the death benefit provided under subsection(a)(2) "in the event of a vaccine-related death."[2]

So the question of whether an estate is limited to only the amount of the death benefit or whether they can receive compensation for emotional distress, pain and suffering, and medical expenses was answered in 2008 by the Federal Circuit Court of Appeals in the favor of the petitioner.

Graves v. HHS

As bizarre as the debate over how and when to award the death benefit is, it is even stranger to determine the logic of how the courts and special masters determine pain-and-suffering awards. To better understand how the calculations for pain-and-suffering are formulated in cases, a review of *Graves v. HHS* is in order.

A petition was filed in September of 2002 claiming that the second dose of the Prevnar vaccine received by the little girl on August 10, 2000, caused seizures. The child passed away on September 24, 2000. An autopsy was performed a few days later, and the pathologist reported that she "died as a result of hypoxic encephalopathy that reportedly occurred following a seizure that developed following a meningitis vaccine."[3] The respondent's own medical expert, Dr. Virginia Anderson, essentially agreed with these findings.[4]

However, the respondent filed a motion to dismiss the petition because the petitioner could not file a report from a medical expert who would testify or submit a medical opinion that the vaccine caused the little girl's death.[5] It took the family several years to finally obtain medical experts who would file medical opinions on the behalf of their daughter. Several hearings were conducted with testimony, medical opinions, and associated literature submitted on behalf of both the petitioner and the respondent.

The special master published his decision in October 2008, ruling that the petitioner failed to meet their burden of proof for an off-table injury using the established Althen three-prong standard.[6]

The Graves's filed a motion for review with the Federal Court of Claims. Before reaching a decision on the motion, the court remanded the case back to the special master to resolve an alternative theory offered by the petitioner in the original testimony, that Prevnar significantly aggravated the little girl's preexisting seizures so that they became more intense and uncontrollable, leading to her death.[7]

The special master concluded in September 2010 that the preponderance of evidence did not support this alternative theory, thus denying the petitioner's motion for review and supporting the special master's decision to deny compensation.[8] However, it was noted that the medical experts concurred that Prevnar could cause subsequent seizures to increase in duration.[9]

Following the remand decision, a careful review was done of the medical records, expert medical testimony, and research studies that had been presented, and the court concluded that the special master erred in denying compensation.[10]

The court then remanded the case back to the special master for a determination of damages. By now the reader may have trouble following this roller coaster process of decisions, opinions, remands, and appeals. However, this is what happens in many off-table petitions seeking compensation after special masters incorrectly determine the credibility of medical reports or medical experts.

In a published remand decision dated August 2012, the special master determined and awarded compensation to the petitioner for the following three segments[11] based on *Zatuchni v. HHS*,[12] in which the Federal Circuit held that estates are not limited to awards of only $250,000:

1. The first part, an award of $250,000 for the death benefit as outlined in statute.
2. For unreimbursed medical expenses incurred between the date of the vaccination and the date of death of the petitioner. The respondent indicated that they did not object to this award.
3. An award for the emotional distress that the petitioner suffered. The parties extensively disputed this issue. Initially, the parties argued whether the Graveses were legally entitled to any amount. A January 2012 ruling resolved this issue in favor of the petitioner. Thereafter, the parties disputed the amount of compensation for the petitioner's emotional distress. An April 2012 ruling awarded a reasonable award of $60,000.[13]

Upon review, the court examined the issue of whether the special master properly applied a policy of the Office of the Special Masters that limited awards approaching or at $250,000 to cases in which the pain and suffering was at the most extreme in intensity, duration, and cognizance of all vaccine-injured petitioners.[14] The court concluded that the special master applied this policy in error and was not consistent with the statute 42 U.S.C. 300aa-15(a)(4).[15] Because of this error, the court awarded the maximum limit under statute for pain-and-suffering and emotional distress to the Graves estate.

In summary, regarding the calculations of pain-and-suffering in the Vaccine Act, damages in the NVICP are typically split into categories for past and future damages.

Future damages, i.e., lost wages and pain-and-suffering, are adjusted to present value. Under the Vaccine Act, pain-and-suffering is capped at $250,000. Prior to the Federal Court of Claims' decision in *Graves v. HHS*, the court interpreted the statutory cap to mean that whatever pain-and-suffering demand a petitioner made it would have to be no greater than $250,000, and the amount would have to be split between past and future pain-and-suffering.[16] For example, a demand of the full $250,000 for P&S would be made as $200,000 for the past and $50,000 for the future—thus maximizing the petitioner's compensation amount, as only the $50,000 in future P&S would be adjusted (reduced) to present value.

The Federal Court of Claims in *Graves v. HHS* held that there is no requirement to split pain-and-suffering into the past and future.[17] Petitioners simply made their total pain-and-suffering demand (using accepted methods, e.g., similar determinations in civil litigation) without regard to the $250,000 statutory cap.[18] If the petitioner's past pain-and-suffering met or exceeded $250,000, or if the petitioner's past pain-and-suffering combined with the reduced future amount met or exceeded $250,000, the special master should award the full $250,000 allowed by the statute.[19]

So we have now established that an estate or representative of a petitioner who died as the result of a vaccine, having proven that the preponderance of evidence clearly states that the vaccine caused their death, can be compensated for the death benefit up to $250,000.00, and also for pain-and-suffering, emotional distress, medical expenses, and in certain cases, loss of future earnings.

This long journey to a fair and just outcome was caused by the vague language about compensation of pain-and-suffering, loss of earnings, and emotional distress within the original act. Like all legal decisions that are precedential in nature, decisions from cases previously adjudicated cannot be reopened. Families prior to Graves cannot retroactively file for additional compensation.

What follows are stories from a few families that had to deal with the loss of their child. The reader will have to decide whether the program is fair and compassionate and whether it creates an overly adversarial process. The reader will have to evaluate whether the government is seeking ways to deny compensation by introducing unbelievable explanations to cloud the reality of vaccine-induced death. What is undeniable is that these families have suffered tragic losses and that the program is re-injuring those seeking closure.

What follows leaves one questioning the government's conduct and the value it places on life.

To Erica

Timothy and Joanna Sarver welcomed their newest family member, Erica, on March 5, 2005. Born with a twinkle in her eye, she was the darling of the household with two older siblings.

High school sweethearts, the Sarvers began a family early and were content with creating a loving and warm home for all, including the newest addition to the Sarver family. But that changed a year later.

Erica was scheduled for her MMR vaccination on March 9, 2006. It was nearly a week after the vaccination when Erica suffered a grand mal seizure. Timothy was at home at the time, noticed what was happening to Erica, and drove her two hours to the ER. Living in rural Iowa, a long drive is often the case for many families. Waiting for an ambulance and then a trip to the hospital would have taken twice as long.

At the hospital, Joanna met her daughter and husband. Both were scared and confused as to what was happening to their beautiful little girl.

Erica was having a series of seizures and they could not be stopped. The doctors, not knowing what was causing these seizures, decided to air flight Erica to Des Moines, to Blank Children's Hospital.

At Blank, the pediatricians and neurologists could not stop the seizures. They also noticed that Erica was going into organ failure, specifically her liver.

Joanna was approached by a friend, who was a nurse. She was aggressive in suggesting Joanna demand that the doctors report this as being a result of the MMR vaccine. But the medical staff assigned to Erica did not accept that her medical condition was the result of a vaccine.

Erica's pediatrician back in Ames, Iowa, contacted the family and suggested that Erica's medical condition could be the result of a vaccine injury. As Joanna discussed this with the pediatrician, she thought only doctors could report such reactions or injuries from vaccines. Joanna remembered receiving a piece of paper (later to be determined to be the VIS) at the moment that Erica received her MMR vaccination. This process did not leave Joanna any time to read or to think about any risks that were associated with this vaccine.

As Erica was fighting for her life at Blank Children's Hospital, the doctors decided on day two to air flight her again. This time it was to Omaha, to a specialized children's hospital for organ failure and possible transplant.

Arriving in Omaha, Erica and Joanna were welcomed by the medical team that was dedicated to saving Erica's life and to find out what had happened to this little girl.

However, the doctors and specialists at the hospital quickly ruled out that any vaccine could have done this to Erica. The Infectious Disease team, which was assembled to help, also ruled out vaccination. How they ruled out vaccination as the source of Erica's medical condition is a mystery.

As the seizures continued and as Erica's liver continued to decline, the doctors placed Erica in a medically induced coma. This was March 22, 2006, nearly one week after Erica suffered her first grand mal seizure. Erica continued to have her blood pressure and heart rate jump up and down. Doctors started to monitor her brain swelling. It appeared to be a dire situation for Erica and her parents.

She started to show signs of stabilizing. Soon, her condition started to improve. And no one could offer an explanation, except for her mother, Joanna, who said that "this was Erica fighting back with the grace of God." Within a few weeks Erica was discharged, and the family returned home to Iowa.

Erica's pediatrician in Ames, Dr. Swanson, contacted the family and suggested that since he believed the MMR injured Erica, they should consider filing a petition with the Vaccine Court to seek compensation for Erica's injuries.

Joanna started to research the NVICP and began to contact attorneys who had represented families. After trying a few who would not answer or return calls, she contacted David Terzian, a Richmond, Virginia–based attorney. Mr. Terzian was once an attorney representing the federal government in opposing petitioners such as Erica Sarver. The stars were aligning themselves, as Mr. Terzian would bring some valuable experience in dealing with vaccine injury petitions, allowing families to feel that he would handle the difficult process and journey.

The petition was filed May 17, 2007, and sought compensation for Erica's pain and suffering, lost wages, past medical bills, and future medical expenses. Once the petition was filed, the Sarvers were relieved that their case was being handled by one of the top attorneys; they also had no reservations about filing. And Erica was improving every day.

However, the constant care that Erica needed demanded that Joanna spend all her time with her daughter, and the attention given to her other children dramatically decreased.

Joanna contacted Iowa's DHS to seek nursing care for Erica. Within a couple of weeks, a case worker for DHS was able to arrange for nursing care. As Erica continued to improve, Joanna turned her time to helping the attorney collect all the necessary medical records and other documentation.

Within three months of filing the petition, they received notice that the court would stipulate damages and move into filing a Life Care Plan (LCP) for Erica. Mr. Terzian contacted a life care planner that he had worked with before to prepare a detailed list of anticipated medical expenses and associated costs for a plan of care for Erica, anticipating that she would live to a normal life expectancy.

The life care planner discussed some difficult issues with the Sarvers to plan for the worst-case scenario. For most of us, trying to plan for what we will need next week or next month is difficult. Now try to estimate all medical costs for the rest of a child's life. A life care planner who is experienced and knowledgeable in this area is priceless.

It became apparent that the respondent's choice for creating a life care plan for Erica was going to be adversarial. Erica's attorney wanted to be present and record all discussions with the government's designee for developing the life care plan. It is a citizen's right under the Seventh Amendment to have counsel present, and Erica's attorney, knowing the history and dealings of government LCPs, wanted to make sure that Erica's interests were represented properly.

Mr. Terzian asked the special master for a ruling. But the special master did not respond nor did they make a ruling on this matter. So instead of this petition moving forward quickly, a stall was the order of the day.

The government life care planner would not file a plan as directed by the court and kept requesting an extension. The special master refused to rule on the matter of recording the proceedings of any discussions or meetings with Erica, her parents, or her doctors, and thus prevented this petition from moving forward. As weeks and months dragged on, the most unfortunate event happened.

Little Erica, still fighting to improve each and every day, made a quick turn for the worse and passed away in December 2008. There was no struggle or pain that Erica faced the last few moments; she just quietly decided it was time.

The Sarvers were now faced with a lasting and impressionable memory of Erica, the little girl who told all the medical doctors a year ago that she was not ready to give up, that she was willing to keep fighting, to keep standing her ground, against all medical explanations when it appeared to be dire.

This family, as several others have done, has had to contend with the death of a child, and has still continued to fight for the petition in Vaccine Court. The process has not been easy. Many families have just given up and moved on. Some keep going. But something was different with the Sarver family. Erica did not give up when she was faced with the worst, so her family decided to continue and not give up.

The petition of *Erica Sarver v. HHS* was finally resolved nearly three and half years after filing the petition in the NVICP. Big delays in this process occurred with the life care planner for the respondent. Maybe they were delaying the process, to wait the family out, making them anxious to resolve this matter and more willing to commit to a lesser compensation award than what the injuries demanded.

Most of the petitions filed in the NVICP for injuries or death are the result of the direct administration of a vaccine or vaccines. However, in a few cases the injured party can be diagnosed with a disease such as polio or influenza as a result of viral shedding.

Gregory Clifford

This next story is about the sad tragedy of Gregory Clifford and his death by viral shedding of the polio vaccine from his baby daughter. His daughter received the oral polio vaccination in May and July of 1998. While not driving trucks, Gregory would be home with his daughter in Texas. Often he would be changing the diaper of his daughter.

A couple of months later, in September, he checked himself into an emergency room at a local hospital claiming leg weakness and suffering acute back pain that had lasted for several days. The following day, he was unable to move his legs. Within two more days, he suffered paralysis of his stomach, respiratory system, and upper extremities.

Three days after arriving in the emergency room, Mr. Clifford suffered respiratory failure and had to be put on a ventilator. The next day, the doctors started to talk with his family about poliomyelitis. A week later, a tracheotomy tube was inserted. Mr. Clifford would remain hospitalized in several different facilities for over a year with no signs of any improvement.

One year later, Gregory Clifford died due to respiratory failure secondary to pneumonia that was caused by paralysis from the polio virus infection. His wife, Holly, filed a petition with the NVICP in July 2001 claiming the death of her husband was the direct result of shedding of the polio vaccination from her daughter to Gregory.

In October of 2001, the respondent (HHS Secretary) filed a report with the special master conceding liability and asking for the special master to award $250,000 for the estate of Gregory Clifford.[20]

What is unknown to most is that the Cliffords have incurred several hundred thousand dollars in medical bills for the care provided to Gregory. These unreimbursed medical expenses needed to be paid. To the respondent, all the petitioner is entitled to is the death benefit and nothing more. Their concern is not for the family that must live without a father and a husband. Their concern is not for the family that must repay thousands of dollars in medical bills that will dramatically exceed any compensation received by the court. Their concern is not about paying for the burial expenses. There is no compassion for the family and no concern for the family's future.

In 2002, several years before *Zatuchni v. HHS* would allow petitioners to seek additional compensation up to and beyond the death benefit, Mrs. Clifford filed an amendment to her petition, arguing for compensation not only for the death benefit, but for the pain and suffering that Gregory endured from the moment he checked into the emergency room in September 1998 till his passing in November 1999, for unreimbursed medical expenses getting close to a million dollars, and for loss of future earnings while hospitalized.

A couple of months later, the respondent filed an objection to the petitioner's request. Thus, the legal maneuvering began. The petitioner, in her request for additional compensation beyond the death benefit, asserted that Gregory Clifford's estate was entitled to additional compensation as stated in the case of *Lawson v. Sec of HHS*. In this case, upon review, Judge Turner ruled that the petitioner could recover damages if they could prove that they had a vaccine injury, but then narrowed his decision to a cap of $30,000.[21]

The respondent then asserted that the Vaccine Act is plain spoken about compensation regarding vaccine injury versus vaccine-related death. They argued that petitioners can only seek unreimbursed medical expenses, pain and suffering, and lost earnings for those with vaccine-related injuries. Vaccine-related death claims can only seek up to $250,000.[22] They found in *Sheehan v. Sec of HHS* that Judge Tidwell held that the Vaccine Act did not permit any award for a vaccine-related death above the amount of the benefit except for additional award of attorney fees.

An interesting note to insert here is that the Vaccine Act of 1986 did not include a provision for unreimbursed expenses. However, in 1983 and in 1984, in failed attempts to pass similar legislation, Congress did include provisions for compensation for medical expenses. The special master in her deliberations of *Clifford* concluded that "Congress may not have contemplated the statute for adult vaccines, who are wage-earners, when it enacted the death benefit statute nor envisioned where a vaccine had prolonged hospitalization before dying from a vaccine injury. However, a petitioner or administrator of an estate can seek remedy in civil courts in those cases in which economic loss and medical expenses far exceed the statutory death benefit."[23] But that option is no longer available in today's setting, after *Bruesewicz* in February 2011.

On July 30, 2002, the special master issued a ruling that the estate of Gregory Clifford was to be awarded the death benefit of $250,000 plus legal fees. It would be a few more years before the NVICP and the legal proceedings decided that families who have lost a husband, wife, son, or daughter can receive compensation for medical expenses, pain and suffering, and loss of future earnings.

Megan

This is the story of a college student, Megan, and her tragic death, as well as of her mother, Karen, and her sisters, who believe that Gardasil led to her untimely death. It was Megan's sisters who witnessed the horrible symptoms she experienced, and the rise of a strong advocate, her mother, who wanted to help prevent more injuries and deaths from Gardasil.

Megan was college bound, ready to embark on becoming a radiologist. She was living with her older sister, Shanna, close to her college. Megan's younger sister, Cara, was also attending the same college.

Megan was the cautious one of the three sisters, conscientious of her own health. It was the fall of 2007 and her doctor told her about Gardasil, how wonderful the vaccine was, and how it was going to prevent cervical cancer. Megan wanted to know more before making a decision. She asked Shanna about the human papilloma virus vaccine. She had seen all the advertisements on TV and read about the many hyped benefits in magazines. Shanna felt that it would be a good thing; it defends against cervical cancer, after all.

Megan later returned to her doctor to start a series of three injections of Gardasil. The first series was administered in the fall of 2007. She started having fainting episodes when taking showers. Her sisters started to notice she was also having headaches and started complaining about extreme fatigue. On one occasion, she told her mom she did not know why she was so tired. She went to bed early, and when she got up in the morning she would have to lay down and sleep for a few hours. Karen kept thinking that all this was due to her new schedule, classes, working, and never connected the dots.

Megan received the second in the series during the spring of 2008. The fainting continued, but depression also entered the equation. Her doctor prescribed an antidepressant. She did not take it as she was scared to take any medication. What her doctor failed to do is connect the dots with her fainting, the depression, the fatigue, and Gardasil. Also, Megan complained to her sisters about having severe headaches and stomach pains, symptoms she had never told her mother about.

In September 2008, Megan received the third and last in the series of Gardasil vaccines. Also at this time, according to her mother, she was having some difficulty dealing with reading and writing comprehension. Megan had begun college and was having to do a lot of essay writing. She would email the essays to her mom and ask for her help as she just couldn't understand what she was writing. Her mother would look at the essays and couldn't understand why she was having such a difficult time. They were so simple.

One afternoon she called her mother to complain of a rash she had all over her face. She had shown her younger sister and told her it was embarrassing. But Megan did not tell her mother about the terrible and extreme stomach pains that she was having. At one point, she called her boyfriend to take her to the emergency room.

It was November 2008 when Megan's boyfriend found her collapsed in the shower. She had passed away sometime that morning while getting ready to go her parents' home to help them paint.

Now a strange and twisted journey to unravel the last days of Megan's life began. Karen was called to the home along with the rest of the family. No one could believe what had happened.

After performing an autopsy, the pathologist could not make a ruling for the reason for Megan's death. They found no water in her lungs, so she did not drown, and the toxicologist report was clean. The official cause of death for Megan is "undetermined."

Weeks passed, and Karen approached Megan's doctor to ask for her medical records. The doctor told her that she would find out what happened and asked if Karen could get all of Megan's previous medical records.

But Karen needed a court order to be awarded the position of executor of Megan's estate. She got a local judge to sign an order and then presented this to the clinic. The clinic replied that they could not hand over the records to her directly, that they must mail them to her. But follow-up phone calls and inquiries to the whereabouts of the records did not produce any results. According to Karen, this seemed to be a stall by the clinic. It took several weeks to receive the medical records. And they did not come directly from the clinic; they came from the office 1,500 miles away in Georgia.

Karen started to research Gardasil and found many families in the state of New Mexico that reported deaths or injuries. She even found another family local to where her daughter had died. The official cause was listed as "undetermined."

Karen approached the Medical Investigator's (MI) office and was told that they would look into the matter. At first, it appeared that the official was looking into Gardasil as the reason for the death of Megan; they sent information to the CDC, but the official was never heard from again.

The MI office also made a request for Megan's medical records. They received them within a couple of days, directly from the hospital. This got Karen curious as to why she had to wait several weeks and then received them from another company.

She also noticed that the medical records she had compared to the records obtained by the MI office were different. There were several missing documents in Karen's copy. But both sets appeared to be incomplete, and they did not contain any record of the third administering of Gardasil.

The official at the MI office stated they did not believe that Gardasil was the cause of Megan's death, nor could they determine what the cause of death was, only that it could not have been Gardasil. Now, where have we heard that before? There is no correlation of vaccines causing autism or other medical conditions, but we do not know what is causing autism.

Karen also wanted to make sure that the rest of the family did not have some form of genetic heart defect or disorder, so they all had themselves checked out by doctors. There were no issues with the rest of the family, so they could rule that out.

Karen talked with a Gardasil injury advocate, and a simple question was asked of Karen: "How many people do you know who are dropping dead of cervical cancer?" Karen replied, "I do not know of any."

That right there got Karen pointed in the direction she is heading now. She started to research Gardasil, finding many families who had suffered similar experiences. Karen contacted the FDA about the dangers of Gardasil and discussed the vaccine with her legislators. She became entrenched in finding out what had happened to her daughter and also in trying to prevent this from harming others.

She was told by friends, neighbors, and others to move on with her life, but she could not. To a mother, it is extremely hard to do this knowing that your child has died and not knowing what caused it. Even today, Karen goes to bed thinking about Megan and wakes up thinking about her heart having a big hole, and that is what is driving Karen to advocate against Gardasil.

During her research, she discovered the NVICP. She contacted a local law firm about her daughter's death. She was told that they were looking into this matter since they had been contacted by as many as seventeen other families who claimed their daughters had died or been severely injured because of Gardasil. Unfortunately, the law firm could not pursue any further action due to the inability to find medical experts to come forth and provide them with medical proof. So, quickly, the law firm contacted all the families and told them that there was nothing they could do for them. This was probably a law firm that knew about the NVICP but wanted a class action law suit, not individual cases.

Even Erin Brockovitch came to town with her team and tried to figure out why there was a Gardasil cluster in Albuquerque, New Mexico. She apparently could not figure it out either and left town quickly.

Karen continued to look for attorneys who would be interested in taking her case. She made many calls and eventually found Mark Sadaka, an attorney with a lot of experience dealing with Gardasil cases in the Vaccine Court. She liked his manner and felt comfortable with what he was telling her about the petition process.

Mark also knew that there were many problems with this vaccine, and he had tried hard to prove that. After filing a petition in June 2010, Karen and her attorney worked to gather the necessary medical records and other documents.

The hospital proved to be the greatest burden in obtaining medical records. Karen remembered Megan receiving the third Gardasil vaccine, yet the hospital showed no records. Megan's boyfriend drove her to every doctor's appointment, and he said that she definitely received the third Gardasil vaccination in September 2010. There was a conversation between Karen and a friend who worked in the billing department of the hospital. Her friend told her that she saw an invoice for the third Gardasil vaccine, yet the hospital records that were produced a few months later mysteriously did not have that vaccine in the medical record.

HIPPA prevented her friend from providing this information to Karen since she was not the legal guardian or executor of Megan's estate at the time.

In March of 2011, fifteen months after filing the petition, Special Master Golkiewicz conducted a hearing in Albuquerque that included questioning from the special master, their attorney, and the DOJ attorney representing the government, along with the entire family and Megan's boyfriend.

During the hearing, the family members were separated and were not allowed to listen to or participate in the other family members' oral testimony. A long and grueling day was ahead. Special Master Golkiewicz approached the entire family afterwards, sat with them, and thanked them for allowing the court to come to their hometown and conduct the hearing. Karen thought that the special master was genuine, courteous, and she felt like he cared deeply about the family and was saddened by the loss of Megan.

However, that would not be the same for the attorney from the Department of Justice. He appeared to be arrogant, not caring about the ordeal that the family was going through, and also seemed to be "put off" that he had to travel to New Mexico to conduct this hearing.

Later that day, after the court officials had left and were returning to Washington, DC, Megan's attorney, Mr. Sadaka, sat down with the family and told them that the hearing did not go well for Megan and that they needed to prepare themselves for having the petition of *Megan Hild (decedent) v. HHS Secretary* dismissed by the court of Federal Claims.

Without a medical doctor to provide expert testimony and with the "lack" of corroborating medical records to prove that Megan had received the third Gardasil vaccination, the special master would have to dismiss the petition. As another attorney who practices in the program told me, Gardasil injuries are autoimmune in nature and are bizarre. From the medical science world, no one can tell you why. No medical expert can testify on what is happening because they do not know why. Gardasil injuries and symptoms are different for each person. And, in the case of Megan, she was slowly deteriorating medically from when she received the first in the series. None of her doctors could connect the dots or look at her medical condition as a whole.

How many more sons and daughters will suffer injuries or die because of a vaccine that was clearly not tested properly? And no one is prepared to determine what will happen to all these girls when they start having children of their own. Karen continues the fight, a strong advocate for others, a voice for Megan. It is "still very important to me to prove that Gardasil took Megan's life."

Chapter 10

Yates Hazlehurst, Michelle Cedillo, and the OAP

How many of us have heard of the Omnibus Autism Proceedings (OAP) and the associated hearings that were conducted in 2007 and 2008? Many can state the names of the first and second petitions that were heard, Cedillo and Hazlehurst. Many in the autism community can tell the general public that the first set of hearings was about establishing the claim that the MMR vaccine and thimerosal-containing vaccines can cause autism. And with great success, many can talk about what Theory 2 and Theory 3 were about: the thimerosal-containing vaccines specifically for Theory 2 and MMR specifically for Theory 3.

By the time the decisions had been published and appeals had been heard for all test cases, there would be nearly 5,500 petitions filed with the NVICP. But the number of hands still up in the air are considerably less when asked what was the name of the petitioner for the third case for Theory 1 (Snyder) and what were the names of the three petitioners for the second theory (Mead, King, and Dwyer).

I tip my hat and congratulate the parents who came forward and volunteered their child's petition as one of the test cases to represent the entire OAP. We are forever grateful for your sacrifice in opening up your family to be inspected by our government and their DOJ attorneys, to become a subject of ridicule and intimidation by those media and medical establishment types who doubt every word and action from you and your family.

A special thank you goes out to all the attorneys who represented the children, for all the long hours, for working seven days a week, all to prepare for the OAP hearings. What most of you have not heard is how the OAP came into existence, the decisions by our government and by a steering committee representing petitioners' attorneys, and how politics, political lobbying, industry heavy-handedness, and personal egos all got in the way of what happened. Nor have you heard that there are many children, thousands of them, some of whom are able to file petitions with the court, most of them who did not, all demanding justice. For many of us, our goal is to study and learn why vaccines can cause injuries or death, and to take steps to prevent the increasing autism epidemic.

I will attempt to guide you through the minefield known as the OAP, introduce several families and share their experiences with you, identify key players within our government that make legal and medical decisions within the OAP, and allow you, the reader, to draw your own conclusions. Maybe after reading and rereading this chapter, you will arrive at the same conclusion that I did while researching this topic. And that is that the OAP, for all the good intentions that it was designed to achieve, quickly became a corrupt legal proceeding, all to accommodate the pharmaceutical industry, the medical community, and our government, instead of determining compensation for thousands of vaccine-injured children and the tens of thousands to come in the future. Get ready, it will be a bumpy ride with a lot of moving parts and flying objects.

The court created the OAP in 2002. Chief Special Master Gary Golkiewicz, from the Office of the Special Masters, issued an order dated July 3, 2002.

> This Autism General Order #1 is being issued by the Office of Special Masters ("OSM") to address an unusual situation facing the National Vaccine Injury Compensation Program ("Program"). This situation arises out of concern in recent years that certain childhood vaccinations might be causing or contributing to an apparent increase in the diagnosis of a type of serious neurodevelopmental disorder known as "autism spectrum disorder," or "autism" for short. Specifically, it has been alleged that cases of autism, or neurodevelopmental disorders similar to autism, may be caused by Measles-Mumps-Rubella ("MMR") vaccinations; by the "thimerosal" ingredient contained in certain Diphtheria-Tetanus-Pertussis ("DTP"), Diphtheria-Tetanus-acellar Pertussis ("DtaP"), Hepatitis B, and Hemophilus Influenza Type B ("HIB") vaccinations; or by some combination of the two.

> When this order was issued, nearly 400 petitions had been filed over the course of two years with the NVICP seeking compensation for vaccine-related injuries that allegedly resulted in autism. Of that amount, nearly 300 were filed in the previous six months.[1]

> Special Master Golkiewicz issued the order out of the developing issue of several hundred petitions filed in the program plus informal discussions held with officials within the Department of Health and Human Services and counsel representing petitioners regarding a decision in the Southern District Court of Texas, *Owens v. American Home Products Corp (2002)*. The ruling stated that all suits against vaccine manufacturers must be filed in the NVICP.

Because of this ruling, attorneys representing several petitioners stated that between 3,000 and 5,000 petitions would be filed with the program in the upcoming months.[2] Needless to say, those numbers would ultimately be correct, but it took a few years instead of a few months. However, in my interview with one of the attorneys I learned that most of the predicted petitioners just gave up. The majority of petitions filed in the OAP would be from new petitioners. So it is quite possible that if the claimants who filed suits prior to the OAP had continued their efforts, the OAP could have been looking at 8,000 to 10,000 petitions instead of 5,500.

In the General Order #1, it is agreed by both parties that the OAP will start to conduct hearings within two years on the general causation. Sometime in the summer of 2004, the evidentiary hearings were to commence.

Then along came *Leroy v. HHS*, a petition filed with the NVICP on April 24, 2002, with a claim that the petitioner received a series of mercury-containing vaccines that caused the child to suffer developmental problems and contesting that the program did not have jurisdiction over this matter. Chief Special Master Gary Golkiewicz issued a Ruling on Jurisdiction on October 11, 2002, in which:

> The petitioner alleges that the vaccine preservative, thimerosal, caused Nicholas's neurologic injury; that thimerosal is not a "constituent material" of the vaccines that he received, "nor does it have any therapeutic effect which would make it a necessary or essential part of any vaccine"; that the Act explicitly excludes thimerosal from coverage because it is an "adulterant" or "contaminant" of the vaccine; that, further, the Vaccine Act never contemplated thimerosal or autism claims; and finally, that thimerosal, because of its toxicity, is not a "constituent material" as defined by the Code of Federal Regulations setting forth regulations for preservatives used in licensed vaccines. For the above reasons, petitioners argue that

any claims alleging injuries arising from thimerosal are beyond this court's jurisdiction. Respondent contends that petitioners' arguments are "without merit" for the following reasons: compensation has been granted to vaccinees for injuries sustained from a vaccine preservative, citing *Grant v. Secretary of HHS*, 956 F.2d 1144 (Fed. Cir. 1992); "thimerosal is neither an adulterant or contaminant within the plain meaning of the Act"; thimerosal is not an adulterant or contaminant when used "within [the] prescribed limits of a valid biologics license"; and, the legislative history supports the proposition that "injuries allegedly related to thimerosal [must] be brought under the Program." Respondent argues further that thimerosal is a constituent of vaccines and the statute makes no distinction between the vaccine antigens and the vaccine's constituent parts. Finally, respondent contends that petitioners' legal position would lead to a "multiplicity of litigation," which is at odds with the Program's legislative purpose.

In their reply, petitioners allege that their claim is not covered under the Program because thimerosal is not a vaccine, but a preservative that "poses a neurotoxic threat to its recipients"; thus, injuries attributable to the ethyl-mercury in thimerosal are not covered. Petitioners also restate that thimerosal is an adulterant and has no therapeutic effect. In this regard, they rely heavily on Special Master Edwards's Order in *Geppert v. Secretary of HHS*, (unpublished Order raising the issue of whether thimerosal is an adulterant or contaminant and directing respondent to file a brief on the jurisdictional issue), for the proposition that injuries from mercury do not fall under the Vaccine Act. They also rely on Magistrate Judge Ashmanskas's recommendation to the federal district court judge in *King v. Aventis Pasteur, Inc.* that a state court could find thimerosal-related injuries are not covered by the Program. See also *King v. Aventis Pasteur, Inc.*, No. 01-1305-AS, Findings and Recommendation, (D. Or. June 7, 2002). Petitioners further contest respondent's reliance on *Grant v. Secretary of HHS*, 956 F.2d 1144 (Fed. Cir. 1992). They aver that the Federal Circuit in that case did not find that the preservative caused the injury, and that Grant is distinguishable because the Leroys' son's injuries were caused by the toxin thimerosal and not by an antigen of the vaccines received, as was the case in Grant. Finally, petitioners contend that irrespective of the Food and Drug Administration's ("FDA") licensing of thimerosal-containing vaccines, thimerosal could not be considered a "constituent material," or component part of a vaccine because it is toxic to the recipient, as evidenced by various agencies' actions.

After considering the parties' arguments, the undersigned finds that subject matter jurisdiction lies properly with this court.[3]

Did you follow that back and forth legal argument? Basically, petitioners could not file claims outside of the program on the basis that thimerosal is not a vaccine. That probably scared the daylights out of the pharmaceutical industry and officials at DOJ and HHS.

Congress would later duplicate this effort by having Senator Bill Frist of Tennessee, whose family owns Hospital Corporation of America, the largest hospital company in the United States, introduce or "sneak" legislation into the Homeland Security Bill of 2002 to prevent lawsuits against manufacturers of thimerosal and forcing any claims against the preservative to be filed within the NVICP.

The year 2002 started out with several developments of major importance: the establishment of the OAP, the Leroy decision on jurisdiction, and Congress sealing the back door. And it is only going to get better or worse, depending on your point of view.

Many have heard of the petition filed in the NVICP in March 2003 by Rolf Hazlehurst and his son Yates. This case, along with

Cedillo v. HHS and *Snyder v. HHS*, would make up the three test cases for Theory 1 of the Omnibus Autism Proceedings (OAP). Theory 1 consisted of the MMR vaccination plus other vaccines containing thimerosal potentially causing autism. The three test cases would represent most of the 5,500 petitions filed with the NVICP, all seeking compensation for vaccine-related injury, including autism.

Theory 2 cases would represent only vaccines containing thimerosal: the three test cases of *King v. HHS*, *Mead v. HHS*, and *Dwyer v. HHS*. Theory 3 cases would represent only the MMR vaccine; however, the Petitioners' Steering Committee (PSC) announced that they would rely on the findings of the cases in Theory 1.

However, most of us do not know about the buildup and legal maneuvering of the first set of hearings in 2007; how a specific petition, *Hazlehurst v. HHS*, was selected to represent a test case; the actual hearings and decisions rendered; and the corruption of the entire process—the manipulation of the process by outside interests, the intimidation of medical experts and petitioners, and how the entire process must not be permitted to happen again.

Yates Hazlehurst was severely vaccine injured and diagnosed with autism at the age of two years, four months. His father, in order to insure that there would be no issue with the statute of limitations, filed the petition just before Yates turned three. The statute of limitations starts the clock upon the first symptom or manifestation of injury. For a majority of the petitions filed in the NVICP that were autism cases and assigned to the OAP, there was the potential they could be excluded by the statute of limitations.

Rolf Hazlehurst, acting upon the knowledge that his son was vaccine injured, started to research the NVICP and attorneys who represent parties that were vaccine injured. Rolf, himself an Assistant District Attorney General for the State of Tennessee, wanted to find someone who practiced vaccine injury exclusively. He desired an attorney with extensive experience with the NVICP.

He found an attorney from Idaho, Mr. Curtis Webb, who has represented many petitioners in the NVICP. However, Mr. Webb did not represent any other petitioners in the OAP. Mr. Webb's extensive experience was representing petitioners who claimed on-table injuries.

In March of 2003, the short-form petition was filed with the court. As with all other petitions that were filed or will be filed with the court claiming vaccines caused autism, they were stayed and transferred automatically into the OAP per Chief Special Master Gary Golkiewicz.

The short-form petition was only three pages long and did not require the petitioner to submit all the medical records and other documents like the normal petition for other vaccine-related injuries or death. Those records would be needed later, however; with the automatic stay they were not required upon filing.

In order to better understand how the OAP was designed to "eliminate" any and all petitions claiming vaccination caused autism, and how the test cases would be set up to be the instrument by which to deny compensation, in this chapter I will provide you with the story of Yates Hazlehurst's petition within the NVICP, the hearing of *Michelle Cedillo v. HHS*, the first test case, and the parallel development of the OAP.

The Omnibus Autism Proceeding was formed July 3, 2002.[4] Special Master George Hastings was selected to preside over the proceedings. In addition, Special Master Hastings was also assigned responsibility for all of the individual program petitions in which it was alleged that an individual suffered autism or an autistic-like disorder as a result of MMR vaccines and/or thimerosal-containing vaccines.[5] The individual petitioners in the vast majority of those cases requested that, in general, no proceedings with respect to the individual petitions be conducted until after the conclusion of the OAP concerning the general causation issue.[6] The plan was that the Office of the Special Masters would deal specifically with the individual cases once the OAP concerning the general causation issue had concluded.[7] If an individual petitioner had their own proof of causation and wanted to "opt out" of the OAP, the petitioner would be allowed to do so.

Later, the Petitioners' Steering Committee (PSC) held telephone conferences to establish procedure for how to conduct hearings for the petitions that were ultimately placed inside the OAP. The PSC is the committee of attorneys representing the petitioners in the OAP. The original hearings were scheduled for March 2004. Special Master George Hastings, in his order of January 2004, reluctantly delayed the hearings until various discovery issues from both sides were resolved.

The PSC would also ask for discovery of certain documents and other materials. Discovery motions generally are not allowed in the NVICP. "There shall be no discovery as a matter of right."[8] Generally, the special master has discretion over the discovery process. Congress intended the program to be quick and efficient. Thus they limited the discovery process. In most civil court proceedings, the discovery process is the issue that creates lengthy proceedings. However, it is a critical process in revealing all facts and the truth.

In the OAP, the parties were encouraged to provide an informal and cooperative exchange of documents and information. The vaccine rules of this court regarding discovery are contained in Rule 7, which provides a special master with the authority to require testimony, or to require submission of evidence or information or documents, "whenever special master deems such testimony, evidence, information, or documents to be reasonable and necessary for the special master's resolution of a vaccine act case."[9] When necessary, the special master, upon request by either party, may approve the issuance of a subpoena. This practice of issuing a subpoena is generally required when one party is having difficulty obtaining necessary medical records or other documentation. All parties are encouraged to provide a cooperative exchange of information; however, if a party feels the informal discovery or cooperative exchange is not sufficient, that party may seek to utilize the discovery procedures provided in the rules of the Court of Federal Claims (RCFC) 26-37 by filing a motion with the court indicating the discovery sought and stating the reasons therefore, including an explanation of why informal practices have not been sufficient.[10] And this would be the route the PSC would follow regarding discovery motions of the Vaccine Safety Datalink.

The PSC filed several discovery motions with the Court. The first motion, filed August 2, 2002, requested materials and documents from several government agencies regarding vaccine injury and vaccine safety and was compiled by the court and delivered to the PSC. The total number of pages of documents provided by the respondent was approximately 218,000 pages. In addition, the PSC was allowed to depose officials from the CDC, the FDA, and the Agency for Toxic Substances and Disease Registry (ATSDR).

The PSC on October 7, 2003, filed a discovery motion requesting Merck & Co., the vaccine manufacturer of the MMR vaccine licensed for distribution in the United States, to provide certain documents. After an evidentiary hearing was conducted in May 2004, Special Master Hastings issued his decision on July 16, 2004, to deny the motion.

On December 8, 2006, a motion from the PSC was filed to compel the respondent to provide documents while seeking access to certain data from the Vaccine Safety Datalink project (VSD). This project is a program sponsored by the CDC in which data is collected from managed care organizations (MCOs) for use in reviewing vaccine safety issues. The VSD includes a large linked database that uses administrative data sources at each MCO.[11] Each participating site gathers data on vaccination (vaccine type, date of vaccination, concurrent vaccinations), medical outcomes (outpatient visits, inpatient visits, urgent care visits), birth data, and census data.[12]

The PSC's experts, through the use of the discovery motion, sought to access the data concerning all children enrolled in all of the eight participating MCOs, approximately 2.3 million children, pertaining to the years 1992 through at least 2004.[13] The desired information includes, *inter alia*,[14] data concerning: all vaccinations received by those children, all diagnoses of those children that fit within one of 35 specific diagnostic codes, the thimerosal content of all lots of vaccine administered after 1999, and all immunoglobulin vaccines or injections administered to the pregnant mothers of those children.[15]

Both the respondent and the MCOs have filed briefs and evidence opposing the PSC's request. They argued that the PSC has failed to show a need for the proposed discovery. They also argued that it would be unreasonable to grant the request, because, they contend, such an order would impose an unreasonable burden on both the CDC and the MCOs and would be contrary to the contractual obligations governing the VSD project.[16] It is quite possible that because of this attempt to provide discovery and access to the VSD, the CDC in the future would alter the structure and the ownership of the VSD to make it virtually impossible for future attempts to access the data.

Special Master Hastings, on January 11, 2007, filed a procedural alteration document to the OAP.[17] He added two additional special masters, Patricia Campbell-Smith and newly appointed Denise Vowell. The selection of Campbell-Smith and Vowell has been met with some suspicion. Why would the court appoint two very newly appointed special masters with less than a few months' experience dealing with vaccine-injury decisions as special masters of the OAP? Campbell-Smith clerked for Court of Federal Claims Chief Judge Hewitt. Special Master Vowell was most recently Chief Army Trial Judge and was part of the Army court that dealt with Abu Ghraib issues. Why were more experienced special masters overlooked? Chief Special Master Gary Golkiewicz, Special Master Abell, Special Master Lord, and Special Master Moran were all available. That question has not been answered and needs to be investigated.

123

The special masters, Hastings, Campbell-Smith, and Vowell, issued a ruling on May 25, 2007, to deny the motion from the PSC for discovery and study of the Vaccine Safety Datalink. In their decision they concluded with the following comments.

First, in reaching this ruling, we are not unmindful of the stakes here. The OAP involves nearly five thousand families with children who suffer from serious and often tragic neurodevelopmental disorders. We are exceedingly sympathetic to the plight of these families. Second, we add that we are not inherently opposed to utilizing the discovery powers provided in the vaccine act to assist these petitioners in obtaining medical records or other materials that may assist them in presenting their cases. To the contrary, and in many of these individual autism cases, we already have, at the request of the individual petitioners, authorized subpoenas so the petitioners could more easily obtain copies of medical records or similar records pertaining to their injured children. Moreover, the record of the OAP demonstrates that, under the supervision of Special Master Hastings, a vast number of documents from government agencies, approximately 218,000 pages, have been supplied to the PSC pursuant to the PSC's initial discovery request. Then, pursuant to the PSC's second round of discovery, the PSC was given substantial access to certain data from the VSD project, enabling experts chosen by the PSC to analyze that data. Accordingly, on an overall basis, one cannot reasonably say that the PSC's discovery requests in the OAP have not met with substantial success. However, after careful analysis of the particular request at issue here, we simply cannot find that the request has merit, for the reasons stated above. Therefore, we have no choice but to deny the request.[18]

It was convenient for the special masters to deny the petitioners access to the Vaccine Safety Data Link. Yet it is the government that relied upon the same system as the basis for their studies that are referenced and cited as evidence in the OAP hearings. This is just another example of the government having access to documents and vaccine safety and injury data and not allowing the petitioners to have access.

On July 18, 2006, the PSC proposed conducting a hearing in June 2007. The original concept of hearings was to conduct them for all the theories of causation. However, on December 20, 2006, the PSC proposed rather than a general causation hearing for all the petitioners' causation theories, the PSC would instead present an actual case as a "test case" to test one of the three general theories; namely the theory that a combination of the MMR and thimerosal-containing vaccines can cause autism.[19] The PSC proposed that the court conduct future hearings on theory 2 of just thimerosal-containing vaccines and theory 3 of MMR only. The court would agree, with the condition that the PSC needed to present two additional petitions for the first set of hearings. *Cedillo v. HHS* would need two additional petitioners.[20] The two petitions needed to be identified to the court by December 30, 1996.

This deadline would not produce the required two additional cases. The court extended the deadline to February 24, 1997, then till March 30, 1997, then to April 30, 1997, and to May 10, 1997. Still no petitions were named by the PSC.

On May 25, 2007, the court issued an Autism Omnibus update to all parties. The court provided an update to the first test case of *Cedillo v. HHS*, scheduled for evidentiary hearings for June 11–26, 2007. In this hearing, the attorneys for both the petitioner, Michelle Cedillo, and the respondent, HHS Secretary, would present testimony for the "general causation issue" of whether the MMR vaccine and thimerosal-containing vaccines can combine to cause autism. Also, the petitioner would present specific testimony on the behalf of Michelle Cedillo, which the PSC selected as the first test case.[21]

The OAP hearings were unique to the court. For previous Omnibus proceedings, a special master would conduct the hearing for a selected test case or cases. In the OAP, three special masters would preside over the hearing. Special Master George Hastings was selected to issue a decision on the specific causation issue over the Cedillo hearing, while the other two special masters would participate in order to hear the general causation evidence.[22]

Also included in the May 25, 2007, Autism Update was the discussion of a "Crisis Point" in the OAP. The court asserted its displeasure with the PSC regarding their inability to find two additional petitions for the upcoming hearings scheduled for June 2007. The court warned that if the PSC and other attorneys that represented petitions assigned to the OAP did not provide two additional petitioners, the court might resort back to adjudicating each petition "case by case," dissolving the OAP, or randomly picking a test case. That would take many years to conduct hearings. This was the extent of the "Crisis Point" segment of the Autism Update of May 27, 2007.

Since the announcement in July 2006 of the proposed hearings to be conducted in June 2007, parents and attorneys, representing the 4,800 petitions, started to prepare and file the necessary medical records, documents, and other information for each petition.

The hearing for the case of *Michelle Cedillo v. HHS* would begin on June 11, 2007, in Washington, DC. The Cedillo family made the trip to Washington, DC, but it took a miracle and a lot of hard work from many people to make it happen. The hearings were scheduled to last two to three weeks. Therefore, the Cedillo family had to make arrangements to live in the DC area for that period of time. There would be no advances of expenses by the court, so the family had to raise the money themselves to "move" from Arizona to Washington for a period of up to three weeks. Michelle's parents had to take another mortgage out on their home to help pay for anticipated expenses.

The hearings would start June 11 with a crowded courtroom at the Federal Court of Claims. Three days prior to the Monday, June 11, 2007, start of the Michelle Cedillo hearing, the respondent announced they would introduce into evidence the Bustin report. The petitioners requested ample time to study the report so they would be able to rebut Dr. Bustin. Special Master Hastings ruled against the petitioner and allowed the respondent to introduce the Bustin report as evidence to discredit the O'Leary labs.

Tissue samples from Michelle Cedillo had been sent to the O'Leary labs for testing. The O'Leary labs confirmed positive measles virus in the gastrointestinal and immune systems of Michelle Cedillo. The O'Leary labs is also the same facility where the twelve tissue samples were collected from children in the Wakefield report, the Lancet 12. So the British government had a severe liability issue with the O'Leary labs. Dr. Bustin was hired by the British government to find evidence and to discredit the O'Leary lab. Bustin was able to cherry pick certain data and evidence to create his own report to discredit the O'Leary labs. So Merck & Co. was able to set the ambush of all the 5,500 petitions filed in the OAP and got Special Master George Hastings to introduce the trap as material evidence.

Also introduced into evidence by the respondent was the medical opinion of Dr. Andrew Zimmerman, a pediatric neurologist from Kennedy Krieger Institute in Baltimore, MD. Dr. Zimmerman has previously been a frequent medical expert for the government. He submitted his opinion in the form of a letter dated April 24, 2007, six weeks prior to the start of the hearing. His opinion was formulated after reviewing medical records of Michelle Cedillo as well as other expert reports filed in this case.[23]

Dr. Zimmerman concluded by stating "there is no evidence of an association between autism and the alleged reaction to MMR and Hg, and it is more likely than not that there is a genetic basis for autism in this child."[24]

What is extremely odd about Dr. Zimmerman is that he was not called by the respondent to appear in person during the trial. And his absence from the witness stand would lead to much speculation about why he was not testifying. And soon we would find out the reason why. It was discovered in another petition that Dr. Zimmerman would reverse himself, concluding that the vaccination did, in fact, contribute to the child's medical condition that ultimately led to the child's autism. And the kicker was that the DOJ attorneys knew of the second opinion from Dr. Zimmerman while they were using his first opinion to prevent compensation for the test cases. This deliberate omission by the DOJ attorneys of key evidence, while protected by the records being sealed in another autism case, would not be allowed in a normal court setting. Yet in the NVICP and specifically the OAP, which procedures are allowed and not allowed is difficult to understand, resulting in an embarrassment for the justice system.

During the hearing, the respondent tried to present a summary of videos of Michelle prior to the MMR vaccination and, with some clever editing, used just a few seconds to try to convince the special masters of specific autistic-like behavior from Michelle. Their effort would fail. Special Master Hastings called Michelle's mother, Theresa, to the stand. Theresa told the court that Michelle did not display any behaviors that would lead a clinician to a diagnosis of autism, which would be obvious if one watched more than a few moments of footage. The respondent would not be finished with this tactic. They would attempt to do the same in other hearings.

During the waning days of the hearings, the respondent called Dr. Bustin from Great Britain to the stand to testify about his report of the O'Leary labs. It would be this report and testimony that would swing the pendulum of justice from the petitioner to the respondent.

Also, legal scholars and attorneys who have practiced litigation in civil court proceedings and the NVICP will tell you that if you enter into evidence a report or study from a medical expert, the expert must testify on behalf of that report. Without the personal testimony, the evidence can be refuted as hearsay and without foundation. Yet in the hearings in the OAP, the special masters allowed this legal proceeding to occur without Dr. Zimmerman's physical presence.

On June 26, 2007, the hearings for *Michelle Cedillo v. HHS* concluded. The decision would not be published for another year and a half. After the grueling twelve-day hearing came to a conclusion, it would take another year before each side was satisfied with corrections of the 2,900-page transcript and nearly five hundred pages of post-hearing briefs and motions.

The Zimmerman report was introduced as evidence against almost every petition filed in the OAP to deny compensation.

Curtis Webb talked extensively with Rolf Hazlehurst about his son's petition. They felt comfortable with the case and documentation: they had all the medical records, CDs containing hours of video, and a medical expert, a pediatric neurologist, ready to testify on the behalf of Yates.

It would be just a couple of days after the issuance of the Autism Update: The Crisis Point Order, that Curtis Webb would receive a call from the special masters asking if he had a petition that was ready to become a test case. Mr. Webb had asked his client, Rolf Hazlehurst, only two weeks prior if he wanted to be named as a test case. Rolf said no. Now the special master was directly asking; Rolf agreed to be the second test case for Theory 1, but only if Yates's neurologist, Dr. Jean-Ronel Corbier, could testify.[25] The PSC had their second test case, just two weeks before the hearing for the first test case, *Cedillo v. HHS*, was to commence.

The PSC had to find one more petition now with Cedillo and Hazlehurst selected. And it was going to get interesting.

In September of 2007, the PSC privately identified the potential test case for the second theory hearings. *Hannah Poling v. HHS* was forwarded to the DOJ and the court as a possible test case. The second theory was regarding thimerosal-containing vaccines allegedly causing autism. The hearings were tentatively scheduled for the last three weeks of May 2008.

The third test case for Theory 1 was announced with *Colten Snyder v. HHS*. This was one of the older petitions, having been filed in 2001. The special master assigned to preside over the hearing would be newly appointed Special Master Denise Vowell. The hearing would commence November 5, 2007, in Orlando, Florida.

In the case of *Hazlehurst v. HHS* and *Snyder v. HHS*, the parties intended to rely upon the general causation evidence presented in *Cedillo*, and the parties authorized the special masters to consider the general causation evidence presented in *Cedillo*.[26] The majority of the hearing would be focused on the specific examination of the individual as they related to the overall theory of MMR vaccine and thimerosal-containing vaccines causing autism. The special masters anticipated that the public participation in the two remaining cases would not be highly attended because of their geographic locations. They would allow the public to attend and would provide recordings of the proceedings in the same manner as *Cedillo*.

The hearings for Cedillo lasted 12 days, which gave Rolf Hazlehurst and his family great pause. But they were eager to finally get their day in court. To prove that Yates was indeed injured by vaccines that he received several years earlier.

The Hazlehurst hearings were conducted over four long days starting October 15, 2007. Since the general causation proceeding was conducted in *Cedillo*, the hearings for *Hazlehurst v. HHS* would focus on the specifics of Yates and his injuries and medical condition.

During the Hazlehurst hearings, the family and their attorney did not know that Dr. Zimmerman had revised his opinion as to the causal link between vaccines and autism or that the Hazlehurst family's testimony about Yates Hazlehurst's constant fever was consistent with one of the critical links in Dr. Zimmerman's revised theory of causation. Basically, he reversed 180 degrees from his position in the *Cedillo* case. But why? The parties would find out a few weeks later.

In his closing argument in the *Hazlehurst v. HHS* hearing, lead DOJ attorney Vince Matanoski argued the following:[27]

> Dr. Zimmerman actually has not appeared here, but he has given evidence on this issue, and it appeared in the *Cedillo* case. I just wanted to read briefly because his name was mentioned several times by petitioners in this matter, what his views were on these theories, and I'm going to quote from respondent's Exhibit FF in the *Cedillo* case, which is part of the record in this case as I understand it:
>
> "There is no scientific basis for the connection between measles, mumps, and rubella MMR vaccine or mercury intoxication and autism despite well-intentioned and thoughtful hypotheses and widespread beliefs about apparent connection with autism and regression. There is no sound evidence to support a causative relationship with exposure to both or either MMR and/or mercury."

According to Rolf Hazlehurst in an interview with this author, it is "inconceivable that the three DOJ attorneys that handled all of the test cases, including *Cedillo*, *Hazlehurst*, *Snyder*, and *Poling*, were unaware that Dr. Zimmerman had revised his opinion. Rolf laid out the timeline for the revision of testimony. Department of Justice attorney Vincent J. Matanoski was the lead trial attorney for all OAP test cases. Dr. Zimmerman was one of the respondent's primary medical experts in the field of child neurology, called upon by the respondent to testify in several previous vaccine-related cases. During the hearing of Cedillo, on behalf of the DOJ and respondent, Matanoski announced to the court that Dr. Zimmerman would not be called upon as an expert witness but rather would just enter his report as evidence. It is obvious to the outside observer that the respondent knew Zimmerman had revised his report but did not want that fact to be known to the petitioner and possibly to the court.

Approximately three week later, on November 9, 2007, the same Vincent Matanoski of the US Department of Justice signed the Rule 4-C report in what would have been one of remaining test cases in the OAP, *Poling v. HHS*.[28] Rule 4-C reports are confidential medical and legal opinions of the respondent outlining the position of whether to compensate a petition or file a motion to dismiss. The specific Rule 4-C report was leaked to the media in March of 2008 and the government's concession to compensate Hannah Poling was now made public. The report contained in part the following:[29]

> In sum, The Division of Vaccine Injury Compensation (DVIC) has concluded that the facts of this case meet the statutory criteria for demonstrating that the vaccinations CHILD received on XXXX [date redacted], significantly aggravated an underlying mitochondrial disorder, which predisposed her deficits in cellular energy metabolism, and manifested as a regressive encephalopathy with features of autism spectrum disorder. Therefore, respondent recommends that compensation be awarded to petitioners in accordance with 300aa-11 (c)(1)(C)(ii).

The government, by conceding the Poling case, prevented Dr. Andrew Zimmerman from taking the witness stand, in which case it could be shown that one expert witness provided two different reports.[30] The first report was used against petitioners Cedillo, Hazlehurst, and potentially all the remaining petitions in the OAP.[31] The second report was used to compensate one child, and in the process the government kept the evidence in her case under seal.[32] "The evidence placed under seal is strong evidence of how vaccines can cause autism."[33] The government fought hard to keep that report under seal and to never allow the public to view the report or know about its existence.

How the government spun the news of Poling concession is a serious case study in itself. HHS hid behind the technical terminology in the Rule 4-C report. What the general public does not understand is that the vaccinations received by CHILD were the MMR and at least one thimerosal-containing vaccine. That was the whole theory of the test cases of *Cedillo*, *Hazlehurst*, and *Snyder*. The government using the phrase "significantly aggravated an underlying mitochondrial disorder" is another way of saying "significant aggravation of a preexisting condition," which is legally a form of causation under the Vaccine Act.[34]

In the Hazlehurst hearing, a 2002 document was introduced as evidence by petitioner, stating Dr. Zimmerman's medical opinion that Yates's neurological condition was "regressive encephalopathy with features of autism spectrum disorder," which is word for word the exact same neurological diagnosis later given to Hannah Poling by Dr. Zimmerman in the government concession in *Poling v. HHS* Rule 4-C report.[35]

According to Rolf, the preliminary medical tests indicated that Yates also had a mitochondrial disorder. To quote Rolf: "The irony is that the stated purpose of the OAP was to determine whether thimerosal-containing vaccines and or MMR vaccines can cause autism and if so, under what conditions was this achieved. However, the government covered up the truth and replaced it with what the government wanted the American people to believe."

On November 19, 2007, the PSC filed with the special masters the first test case for Theory 2, that thimerosal-containing vaccines caused autism. The petition of *William Mead v. HHS* was filed with the NVICP in January of 2003. Thomas Powers, the lead attorney for the PSC, would be the attorney of record for the petitioner. Special Master Campbell-Smith would preside over the proceedings.

Later, the PSC would announce that the petition from *Jordan King v. HHS* would represent the second test case for Theory 2. Special

Master Hastings would preside over the hearing. The last test case for Theory 2 would be *Colin Dwyer v. HHS*. Special Master Vowell would preside over the proceedings.

During a hearing conducted in Washington, DC, on May 12–30, 2008, the parties presented general causation evidence on the second theory of causation and presented specific causation evidence in the *King v. HHS* and *Mead v. HHS* cases regarding whether the thimerosal-containing vaccines had caused the autistic condition of the vaccinated children whose particular cases were being heard.[36]

During another hearing conducted in Washington, DC, July 21–22, 2008, the parties presented more general causation evidence and specific causation evidence in the *Dwyer v. HHS* case.[37]

In April 2008, the parents of Hannah Poling wanted to discuss their child's case with media and the public, thus they filed a motion with the court, "Motion for Complete Transparency of Proceedings." The DOJ and the respondent opposed this motion, and for good reason if they were going to continue to hide from the American public that vaccines can cause autism.

The special master held a status conference call with all parties to address the filed Rule 4-C report. In their motion for transparency, the Polings referred to an expert report from Dr. Andrew Zimmerman (who filed the report against Cedillo and Hazlehurst), Hannah's neurologist, in support of the petitioner's claim that Hannah's complex partial seizure disorder was a result of her vaccine-related injury.[38] The respondent, in her Rule 4-C report, stated that the onset of Hannah's complex partial seizure disorder was not related to her vaccinations.[39]

By conceding the fact of the complex partial seizure disorder, Dr. Zimmerman was still not subject to direct examination on the witness stand, and the record of *Poling v. HHS* remains sealed and confidential.

February 12, 2009

Just two days prior to Valentine's Day of 2009, the special masters released the final decisions of the test cases for *Cedillo v. HHS*, *Hazlehurst v. HHS*, and *Snyder v. HHS*. It would not be a good day for any petitioner. Special Master George Hastings issued his decision to deny Michelle Cedillo compensation, Special Master Patricia Campbell-Smith issued her decision to deny Yates Hazlehurst compensation, and Special Master Denise Vowell issued her decision to deny compensation for Colten Snyder. All three decisions were denied on the basis that the petitioner failed to establish both specific and general causation. For the thousands of families that anxiously waited for the decisions, it did appear that the decisions were orchestrated and that the government got what it wanted from the beginning.

In his decision of *Cedillo v. HHS*, Special Master George Hastings wrote the final three paragraphs to the Cedillo family specifically.

The record of this case demonstrates plainly that Michelle Cedillo and her family have been through a tragic and painful ordeal. I had the opportunity, in the courtroom during the evidentiary hearing, to meet and to observe both of Michelle's parents, and a number of other family members as well. I have also studied the records describing Michelle's medical history, and the efforts of her family in caring for her. Based upon those experiences, I am deeply impressed by the very loving, caring, and courageous nature of the Cedillo family. Those family members clearly have done a wonderful job of coping with Michelle's conditions, and in caring for her with great love. I admire them greatly for their dedication to Michelle's welfare.

Nor do I doubt that Michelle's parents and relatives are sincere in their belief that the MMR vaccine played a role in causing Michelle's devastating disorders. Certainly, the mere fact that Michelle's autistic symptoms first became evident to her family during the months after her MMR vaccination might make them wonder about a possible causal connection. Further, the Cedillos have read about physicians who profess to believe in a causal connection between the MMR vaccine and both autism and chronic gastrointestinal problems. They have visited at least one physician, Dr. Krigsman, who has explicitly opined that Michelle's own chronic gastrointestinal symptoms are MMR-caused. And they have even been told that a medical laboratory has positively identified the presence of the persisting vaccine-strain measles virus in Michelle's body, years after her vaccination. After studying the extensive evidence in this case for many months, I am convinced that the reports and advice given to the Cedillos by Dr. Krigsman and some other physicians, advising the Cedillos that there is a causal connection between Michelle's MMR vaccination and her chronic conditions, have been very wrong. Unfortunately, the Cedillos have been misled by physicians who are guilty, in my view, of gross medical misjudgment. Nevertheless, I can understand why the Cedillos found such reports and advice to be believable under the circumstances.

I conclude that the Cedillos filed this Program claim in good faith. Thus, I feel deep sympathy and admiration for the Cedillo family. And I have no doubt that the families of countless other autistic children, families that cope every day with the tremendous challenges of caring for autistic children, are similarly deserving of sympathy and admiration.

However, I must decide this case not on sentiment, but by analyzing the evidence. Congress designed the program to compensate only the families of those individuals whose injuries or deaths can be linked causally, either by a Table Injury presumption or by a preponderance of causation-in-fact evidence, to a listed vaccination. In this case the evidence advanced by the petitioners has fallen far short of demonstrating such a link. Accordingly, I conclude that the petitioners in this case are not entitled to a Program award on Michelle's behalf.[40]

It would appear that all the research, all the efforts by the Cedillo family were for naught. Special Master George Hastings is entitled to his opinion, one that should be taken seriously, as he presided over the lengthy hearing, reviewed over 930 pages of medical literature, and sifted through approximately 8,000 pages of medical history and documentation of Michelle Cedillo. And those who support the government's position that the MMR did not in fact cause Michelle's autism, and those who also champion the comments of the special master instructing the family that they were misled by a few medical practitioners, started to strut their own sense of relief and "I told you so" attitude.

However, were the special masters misled in the presentation of the evidence, were they hoodwinked about the facts? After reading the 2,900 pages of the oral transcript of the hearing, I arrive at a different conclusion. Granted, I do not have access to the hundreds of pages of medical records and medical expert reports presented during the hearing. I did have access to the family, I did speak with a couple of the medical experts for Michelle Cedillo, and I do have knowledge of the deliberate nondisclosure of key evidence. After all of this research I decided that the conclusion reached by the special masters was a stretch, not a slam dunk, and was far from a decision based upon all the medical evidence.

There are many children in the United States with similar medical conditions as Michelle Cedillo. How did this happen, other than by a vaccination? They all live in different areas of our nation. They are not related to each other. Most of them have brothers or sisters who did not suffer the same adverse reactions. Could it be that the MMR vaccine and/or thimerosal-containing vaccines caused these injuries? What else could it be other than our government, plus the British government, the pharmaceutical industry, health-related media types all defending a product with such zeal, with great effort, sparing no expense, stomping on the life of Michelle Cedillo, Yates Hazlehurst, and Colten Snyder, or the several thousand other children?

Petitioners filed a motion for review with the court one month after the decision. In their March 16, 2009, motion, Cedillo outlined a number of objections.

1. The use of a panel of three special masters to hear "General Causation" issue in Michelle's case was arbitrary, capricious, an abuse of discretion, and not in accordance with the law.
2. The special masters' decision to allow the last-minute expert reports and testimony of Dr. Stephen Bustin was arbitrary, capricious, and an abuse of their discretion.
3. The special master abused his discretion by discounting the opinions of Michelle's treating physicians.
4. The special master abused his discretion by ignoring concessions by the respondent's expert witnesses.
5. The special master abused his discretion by simply ignoring other important aspects of Michelle's evidence.
6. The special master abused his discretion by refusing to consider significant post-hearing evidence.
7. The special master's decision was not in accordance with the law.

In the conclusion of their motion for review, Cedillo requests that she is entitled to compensation and her case be remanded to the special master to assess appropriate compensation.

Oral arguments were heard July 7, 2009. Judge Wheeler of the Federal Court of Claims issued his decision on August 6, 2009, denying the petitioner's motion for review.

Cedillo filed for an appeal of her case to the United States Court of Appeals for the Federal Circuit in October 2009.

In a January 25, 2010, Brief of Amici Curiae,[41] Mary Holland, Esq., writing for the Elizabeth Birt Center for Autism Law and Advocacy (EBCALA) in support of Appellants (Cedillo) and in Favor of Reversal, argued that the Federal Court of Claims failed to criticize the partisan tone of the special master's decision.[42] Do you recall the last three paragraphs of Special Master George Hastings's decision criticizing Michelle's treating physicians and telling Michelle Cedillo and her family that they have been misled, that her doctors were "very wrong," and that her doctors "are guilty . . . of gross medical misjudgment?" The special master's limited role is "to apply the law." His role is not to displace the court of Federal Claims or to chastise the petitioner, her lawyers, or experts. His role is to "aid judges in the performance of specific judicial duties." Special Master George Hastings abandoned this role when he issued his opinions in the final segment of the decision.

On August 27, 2010, the Court of Appeals for the Federal Circuit issued their decision to affirm Special Master George Hastings's decision to dismiss.

But there is so much more to this tragic story of the *Cedillo v. HHS* petition than its just being dismissed—much more. Only a few years later, it appears that we do know our government might have conspired to fix the outcome of the case. What would have happened if Michelle Cedillo had won compensation in the OAP? Would there be mass hysteria, a dramatic decrease in vaccination rates because it was found that the MMR and thimerosal-containing vaccines could cause autism? Would there be a mass rush by hundreds if not thousands more children who claimed a vaccination caused their autism or other disability?

The standard of proving off-table causation is known as the Althen standard, and Michelle Cedillo met her burden of proof under Althen. But yet, the special master ignored this.

The federal government and the respondent in the OAP hearings relied upon epidemiological studies researching infant disabilities, autism, and genetic disorders conducted by the CDC. Many of these studies were conducted in Denmark from 2002 to 2007 under the direction of lead investigator Poul Thorsen. As the lead investigator, Mr. Thorsen's research concluded that there was no link between childhood vaccinations and autism. As Dr. Max Wiznitzer, a frequent medical expert for the respondent, stated in his criticism of another doctor, "If you can't trust the researcher, you can't trust the research." Mr. Thorsen was indicted by the Northern District of Georgia District Court on April 18, 2011, for embezzlement of research grant money for his personal use. Mr. Thorsen is now on the FBI's Most Wanted List and currently is not in the United States. So how much of the research is credible?

There have been a few books written referencing the outcome of *Cedillo v. HHS*. Many interviews were conducted with Pharma-friendly media and journalists, hundreds of papers were written about the virtues of the program. But all have fallen short of reporting the entire story of this case and the remaining petitions scheduled to be heard in the OAP. Most of these articles and books tout the ability of the DOJ attorneys to "tear down" the medical experts for the petitioners. To question their writings, to cast doubt on their comments, is the motive of government counsel. It is to be expected during any cross examination by the opposing counsel.

But what has not been reported by this same group was the possible malfeasance, fraud, and manipulation of evidence by the respondent. To stop Michelle Cedillo from winning in court, the respondent had to cast doubt about the credibility of evidence from Unigenetics Laboratory in Dublin, Ireland, and the clinical report of measles virus in Michelle's body. Dr. Bustin's testimony in Cedillo is focused around the MMR laboratory results of the O'Leary labs and their conclusions that the MMR causes persistent measles in the gastrointestinal and immune systems.

Three days before the commencement of the hearing, DOJ attorneys announce that they would be introducing the Bustin report at trial as evidence to support their claim of the O'Leary lab reports being not accurate. So questions need to be asked. How did the DOJ obtain the Bustin report? The report was to be sealed within the United Kingdom's legal system as part of the UK Litigation of the MMR. Who leaked or allowed the report to be made public? It would be revealed later that our federal government obtained the report only after an extraordinary and expensive multi-month effort without informing the petitioner's counsel.

Cedillo attorneys argued that the report was nothing more than "cherry picking" from many expert reports, that they were not given proper time to prepare to examine or argue the merits or credibility of the Bustin report, and that the actions of the federal government covertly obtaining a report using unlimited financial resources was legally "dirty" business. One ironic issue about this mess is that the PSC had asked Special Master Hastings three years prior to subpoena the same reports from Merck, the vaccine manufacturer, as a defendant in the English High Court cases, known as the UK Litigation.[43] Special Master Hastings would deny the PSC their motion.

The US government was able to obtain the Bustin report at the last minute due to some unexpected help by Merck and their attorneys. And it was a British journalist, Brian Deer, who told the US government that the report existed. Deer even bragged about it in a couple of interviews with certain Internet bloggers. Deer is a central figure in the discussion of how certain confidential medical evidence in British litigation ends up in his hands.

Why is a British journalist involved in an American legal proceeding? It comes down to one person, Dr. Andy Wakefield. For it was Dr. Wakefield who co-authored a paper, published in the *Lancet* in 1998, detailing the case histories of twelve children who developed significant bowel disease from the MMR vaccine and who later were diagnosed with autism. The same Dr. Wakefield authored a 250-page document on the safety of the measles vaccine in 1995 and co-authored a paper published in the *Lancet* in 1995 called "Is measles vaccine a risk factor for inflammatory bowel disease?"

During a press conference called by the Dean of St. Mary's Medical School in 1998, where his co-author, Professor John Walker-Smith, had established his practice as one of the world's leading pediatric gastroenterologists, Dr. Wakefield responded to a question about the safety of the MMR vaccine.[44] He suggested that concerned parents may wish to use single vaccines spaced out—which was then an option on the UK National Health Service, soon to be removed by the government and the vaccine manufacturers in the following months, thus provoking a crisis.

This announcement created a firestorm in the media and medical community of Great Britain. So much so that a few months later, the British government terminated the supply and availability of the single-vial vaccines, presumably from pressure from the pharmaceutical industry, namely Merck. This was not the first time the MMR vaccine's safety was called into question in Great Britain. In 1992, two versions of the MMR from other manufacturers were removed from the marketplace due to claims of being unsafe. The two versions contained the Urabe mumps strain manufactured by SKB, later GlaxoSmithKline and Aventis Pasteur, even later Sanofi.

This created a major health policy concern for the British government, knowing that vaccination rates would plummet as parents decided in favor of vaccine safety instead of vaccination. The British government and the pharmaceutical industry were in a tough spot.

Enter Brian Deer, who has previous work experience writing about medical issues, including trying to discredit an Irish family that received compensation for injuries received from the DPT vaccine. In 2003 he was approached by a *Sunday Times* editor to find something "big" on the MMR. He started to investigate Dr. Wakefield, and in 2004 published a story in the *Sunday Times* (London) detailing alleged undisclosed conflicts of interest. After publishing his article, he sent a letter to the General Medical Council (GMC). This organization is similar to, in the United States, the American Medical Association (AMA).

The GMC started its own investigation. February 8, 2009, Deer published another article accusing Dr. Wakefield of fixing the data in the study that he published in the *Lancet* back in 1998. This article was posted just four days prior to the decisions in *Cedillo, Hazlehurst,* and *Snyder* were to be announced. Coincidence?

Deer, having spent most of the Cedillo hearing trying to chase down the family as they left the courtroom, or trying to catch the same elevator with the family, leads one to suspect that Deer was not there to cover the hearing for a newspaper. He went on US college tours to present his findings and to promote himself as the little reporter that brought down Dr. Wakefield. However, he would not engage in any substantive questioning of his conclusions nor entertain a debate-style format about his investigation. Often a frequent user of curse words in his presentations, he would entertain his audience instead of informing of the facts.[45] Prior to his presentation at the University of Wisconsin–LaCrosse, Brian Deer had the first slide of his presentation displayed on the large screen for all attendees to read as they entered the conference hall. Deer remarked, "If he wasn't so fucking greedy, he'd been tougher to spot."[46]

But how did Deer know about the existence of the Bustin report to begin with, and how was he able to obtain a copy of the confidential report? Did he obtain the report illegally under English law? And if the US government or the DOJ attorneys were informed by Deer that a report existed, would this be considered inadmissible evidence? Generally, documents obtained by a journalist are not admissible. They did receive a document from Brian Deer. But to provide the legal cover, our government officially and quietly without informing petitioner's counsel filed for a copy of the Bustin report and received it just days before the Cedillo hearing.

Multiple sources all report the inappropriate discussions between Brian Deer and the government's expert, Dr. Bustin, during the last days of the hearing. It does appear that Bustin had many things to answer for. Deer, on the other hand, is generally regarded as a hired hit man disguised as a journalist. His direct claim that the case of "*Michelle Cedillo v. HHS* was a fraud" has been refuted, and his investigation and allegations against Dr. Wakefield have been debunked by Dr. David Lewis. Mr. Deer has shown time and time again that his work is not credible and was orchestrated by the *British Medical Journal* and the British government.

A question that needs to be asked of the special masters is the following: It was known that Dr. Bustin received funding by Merck for his research in the United Kingdom. Why did the special masters allow Dr. Bustin to testify in the hearing about a Merck product, the MMR vaccine?

Also, since this hearing had reached full-blown litigation status, how was the defendant able to introduce Dr. Bustin's report without having Dr. Bustin testify? In normal civil court proceedings, a medical expert's report cannot be entered into as evidence unless the medical expert is available for testimony. Otherwise it is treated as hearsay due to the lack of foundation. In the Hazlehurst hearing, the report was introduced as evidence by the lead DOJ trial attorney, Vince Matonoski, yet Dr. Bustin was not compelled to testify by Special Master Campbell-Smith.

My FOIA requests to HRSA, CDC, and DOJ asking for all emails, documentation of correspondence, and other materials provided to each agency from Brian Deer and Dr. Bustin have gone unfulfilled.

* * *

Because the proceedings and rulings in *Poling v. HHS* were sealed, and even though the Rule 4-C report was leaked, these documents could not be used in any future hearings in the NVICP. Thus, these documents cannot be introduced in any appeal proceeding to raise the issue of government misconduct.

After the conclusion of the Hazlehurst hearing and prior to the decision, Curtis Webb filed a motion with the court to strike certain evidence that was introduced in the Cedillo hearing regarding the testimony of Dr. Stephen Bustin from Great Britain. Curtis Webb, the attorney for Yates Hazlehurst, filed a motion to strike the evidence from Steven F. Bustin, on the basis that Hazlehurst was not a party to the UK litigation.

Special Master Campbell-Smith found Yates Hazlehurst's pediatric neurologist, Dr. Corbier, to be very qualified but not persuasive because he was basing his conclusions of what was happening with Yates on the lab results from the O'Leary Lab. Special Master Campbell-Smith found the O'Leary Lab to be not credible because of the Dr. Bustin report, which was introduced in the eleventh hour of the Cedillo case. Attorney Curtis Webb commented that the hearing process for these families had turned into a full-blown product liability litigation instead of what Congress intended to be a fair, quick, and non-adversarial process.

On appeals, the Federal Circuit Court of Appeals agreed that the process of allowing Bustin's report was unfair. But the court's remedy for the unfairness was going to be satisfied by allowing the petitioner to go to England and depose Dr. Bustin and investigate his report. Basically, the court was telling Rolf Hazlehurst that you can go to England and depose the medical expert used in the Michelle Cedillo hearing, but at your own expense. Rolf estimated that cost to be anywhere from $400,000 to $500,000 to properly depose Dr. Bustin and conduct their own investigation of his report.

For someone who had to borrow money to pay for his committed medical expert, Rolf simply did not have the additional funds to travel to England. And under British law, Dr. Bustin was not compelled at all to talk to the American attorneys. So according to Rolf, his case had now morphed into a case of international litigation, having to take on the entire British Empire, by deposing their hired gun medical expert Dr. Bustin. This is the same government that crucified Dr. Wakefield. But there is a question that still remains and that is this: How did the DOJ attorneys who represented the respondent in the Michelle Cedillo hearing get a hold of the Dr. Bustin report?

Hazlehurst quickly filed a motion for review of the special master's decision. This motion would be directed toward the Federal Court of Claims. Petitioners contended that the special master improperly based her decision on evidence that should have been excluded (Bustin), disregarded other evidence that should have been considered, and declined to decide an issue of fact necessary for a reasonable resolution of their claim. Oral arguments were heard in June 2009. Judge Weise issued his decision to deny the petitioner's motion on July 24th.

Later, the case would be appealed to the Federal Circuit Court of Appeals requesting a remand, one step below the US Supreme Court.

Also during the oral arguments in front of the US Federal Circuit Court of Appeals, DOJ attorney Lynn Ricciardella responded to the court's question regarding the emerging scientific and medical evidence of whether vaccines can cause autism by saying, "We're not even at the stage where it's medically or scientifically possible."[47] She stated this to the Court of Appeals judges with full knowledge that she also signed the Rule 4-C report conceding Hannah Poling suffered autism as a result of a vaccine injury and that she was in possession of Dr. Zimmerman's second opinion stating that he was of the opinion that the vaccines caused Hannah Poling to suffer injuries including autism.[48]

On May 10, 2010, the Federal Circuit Court of Appeals issued their decision affirming Special Master Patricia Campbell-Smith's decision to dismiss.

The OAP was supposed to be about conducting hearings, listening to both medical experts and the family members of the children who were vaccine injured, and reviewing medical research in order to reach a logical conclusion as a representative case for the nearly 5,500 petitions filed in the NVICP regarding claims of injuries resulting in autism.

What it actually turned into was a full-blown litigious circus of "gotcha." Looking back, the respondent relied on research and studies from a federally indicted researcher, DOJ attorneys demonstrated blatant use of a medical expert and his report knowing all along that this same medical expert actually issued another report that supported the petitioner's claim, the respondent introduced suspect medical experts and their reports that were sealed in another country's litigation, and the special masters exhibited a partisan tone and many criticisms against doctors and experts—our federal government clearly did not want any petitioner to prevail.

As a result, thousands of children will not have their "day in court." The balance of the petitions in the OAP will be systematically dismissed over the course of the next few years. Parents are left with no faith in a partial and biased judicial system. Many parents have waited five years, eight years, or even longer. They still struggle day to day providing the necessary medical care their child requires.

The following is a story of one mother who continues to fight for her son, having placed her faith in a system that was to determine compensation for her vaccine-injured child.

A Warrior Mom and Her Son, Dayton

You have probably heard a term before—"Warrior Mom," specifically "Autism Warrior Mom." This is a story about a true warrior mom and her son, Dayton.

When Dayton was eighteen months old Kimberly took him to his pediatrician for the MMR vaccine. Within hours of getting the vaccination, Dayton broke out with a rash on the small of his back and developed a high fever. Even though doctors mention it is possible for children to break out with a fever after vaccines, this was the first time Dayton ever did. At first, Kimberly didn't make the connection

that this could be the result of a vaccination. Dayton was also playing outside with some children the day he received his MMR and
she thought possibly the rash was from the grass or weeds. After
researching on the Internet, she thought Dayton might have contracted chicken pox.

Also, Dayton was speaking at the time of his vaccination but
immediately lost his language after receiving it. He seemed quite dis-
tant and off in his own world. Dayton began rocking and flapping
his hands. Kimberly was extremely worried but still uncertain of the
cause of this change of behavior in her son.

But something else happened to Dayton. He had fallen and bitten
his tongue, which required stitches days after his MMR. Kimberly
wanted to believe Dayton's tongue wound was the reason for his
loss of language. Kimberly thought that this is the reason why he
didn't talk anymore. He was trying to nurse back his tongue that
had several stitches, but it continued for a few weeks. Kimberly
started to research by reading articles from the Internet about loss
of language and rashes.

She started to look at other possibilities. Was Dayton injured
because of the vaccination? First, she had his hair follicles checked
for mercury. She had read a few articles regarding the live virus
remaining in certain children, so she next had his colon scoped, and
that is where she discovered the live MMR virus was still present in
Dayton.

From there she started reading about biomedical interventions
to help improve his gastrointestinal system and his immune system,
but Dayton still had severe behavioral issues. It wasn't long before
Kimberly figured out that Dayton was vaccine injured. However, she
wasn't ready to accept it. She did not want to believe it.

Once Kimberly accepted Dayton's injury in the cause, she spoke
with her father, who is an attorney. He started to explore the legal
options for Kimberly and then contacted a few attorneys who possibly could help his grandson. Kimberly started attending conferences

around the country, including Autism 1, and became active in discussions with Talk About Curing Autism (TACA).

Her father contacted an attorney in New Jersey, a Mr. Thomas Gallagher. After months of researching and accepting the fact that Dayton was vaccine injured, Kimberly then called Mr. Gallagher to start the process of filing a petition in the vaccine court. He was courteous and showed compassion toward the family. She was told to send medical records to the attorney as soon as possible. The National Vaccine Injury Compensation Program had already started to identify over 5,000 petitions claiming vaccine injury that caused autism.

Her petition was filed in August 2005. The petitioning families soon received a notice from their attorneys that this process had been put on hold. The Omnibus Autism Proceeding (OAP) would not start until two years later, in 2007. And Dayton still needed care and medical services.

However, Kimberly did receive a few status updates from her attorney as she helped in obtaining medical records and other documentation for Dayton's petition.

As is the case with many of the petitions, the stability of the family was being severely tested. Unfortunately for Kimberly, in addition to finding qualified therapists and providing care for Dayton, she also had to deal with her divorce proceedings. She was also going to school and working. She did not attend the OAP hearings but was following along with daily updates. Kimberly was very optimistic about the hearings, for she had to believe in something.

As initial OAP proceedings wound down, she was disappointed in the hearing outcome. As busy as she was, she let her father update her on the status of her petition. She chose not to think about it in order to concentrate on her son, her school, and work.

As with over 5,400 other petitions, Dayton's was dismissed in October 2011. She found this out by talking with a few advocates who were monitoring the OAP and the subsequent dismissals.

Looking back, she had been hopeful that Dayton's petition was going to succeed. She'd felt confident, especially as she had ruled out all other possibilities as to why her child developed these severe behavioral issues. It was not normal or genetic; she saw the dramatic decline in his overall health, starting with the eighteen-month MMR vaccination.

But as with many people who deal with disappointment or tragedy, new opportunities are born, a door is opened, a new chapter starts—she decided to take advantage of this new episode in her life.

She focused her education around becoming a national board-certified behavioral analyst and currently is working to open an autism therapy day school in her home state of New York.

Chapter 11

Is It Genetic or Is It Vaccination?

As the battle rages on between petitioners filing claims of vaccine-related injury or death and the government always denying any injury or death was the result of vaccination, another trend is developing within the NVICP. For the last couple of years, the media has flooded the print and video worlds with stories about how "It's the parent's age that causes autism,"[1] or about studies that assert "the association of gene mutation with increased risk of conditions like schizophrenia or autism."

Now comes the advancing position defended by the courts, DOJ attorneys, and the HHS Secretary, which is that seizures that occur after the DTaP vaccination are caused by the SCN1A gene mutation or Dravet Syndrome instead of the vaccination. A pattern of denial of vaccine injury has also emerged.

In 2006, Dr. Samuel Berkovic of the Epilepsy Research Center at the University of Melbourne, Australia, published a study entitled "De-Novo Mutations of the Sodium Channel Gene SCN1A in Alleged Vaccine Encephalopathy: A Retrospective Study."[2] The small case study of fourteen patients concluded that the onset of seizures or seizure disorders occurring after the administration of vaccination was the result of the underlying medical condition of the SCN1A gene mutation and not the result of the vaccination.[3] Then Dr. Paul Offit, a prominent vaccine proponent and an avid spokesperson for the vaccine industry, based upon this one small case study, concluded the following: "Individuals who developed their seizures within seventy-two hours of vaccination would have developed their seizure disorders in any event because of their genetic mutation in the SCN1A gene."[4]

Dr. Anne McIntosh published a paper "to establish whether the apparent association of Dravet Syndrome with vaccination was caused by recall bias and, if not, whether vaccination affected the onset or outcome of the disorder."[5] The interpretation of the outcome of the study concluded that "vaccination might trigger earlier onset of the Dravet Syndrome in children, who, because of an SCN1A mutation, are destined to develop the disease. However, vaccination should not be withheld from children with SCN1A mutations because we found no evidence that vaccination before or after disease onset affects outcome."[6]

In an accompanying commentary to the McIntosh study, one of the hired medical experts for the government, Dr. Max Wiznitzer, said, "McIntosh's study was consistent with the conclusion that outcome is determined by the underlying disorder and not by proximity to vaccine administration."[7]

So the obvious question here is, if it is indeed the gene mutating, then how does the body know when the child will receive the vaccination? It does not, and the conclusion is absurd on several fronts, such as:

1. the conclusion that eleven out of the fourteen children had the gene mutation, which is not a proper medical foundation to state that all seizures as a result of vaccination are the result of the gene mutation;

2. according to the McIntosh study, vaccination can trigger an earlier onset of Dravet Syndrome, but has anyone else noticed that seizures and seizure disorders at a very early age are more damaging to the brain development than later in life? Perhaps vaccines should be delayed to allow more brain development;

3. while there remains a possibility of causation in some circumstances, large population-based epidemiological studies are required before concluding that vaccines played no role or even no aggravating role in the onset of such catastrophic symptoms;[8]

4. this case study, along with the McIntosh study, provides the HHS Secretary and the DOJ attorneys the ammunition they need to defend their position that vaccines do not cause seizures, seizure disorders, and epilepsy;

5. the government's position, that if you have SCN1A, you will have seizures, has not been proven—little science exists to support that position; and

6. the common statement from DOJ attorneys and their medical experts used to base their legal or medical opinions on, "the child will suffer seizures anyway," is ridiculous at best and is not based on credible research or science. It even suggests that the respondent does not consider the petitioner, the young child suffering from seizures and epilepsy, as a human being, but rather as a lab rat or some collateral damage that is necessary for the greater good.

The important take-away from the Macintosh study is that the authors concluded that there was no rational basis for withholding the DTaP immunization "for fear of causing Dravet Syndrome or entering the brain by direct or presumed immune mediated mechanism." So is that the rationale our government is making the determination that if a child has Dravet Syndrome it is the sole cause of the seizure disorders and epilepsy episodes? And according to the McIntosh study, they conclude that it does not matter whether or not the vaccine triggered an earlier onset of Dravet Syndrome, as "they are going to get it sooner or later."

In January 2014, the compensation awards of both *Jordan Harris v. HHS* and *Ned Snyder v. HHS* were overturned by the Federal Circuit Court of Appeals. In both cases, petitioners were awarded large compensable damages for their vaccine-related injuries—both were administered the DTaP vaccine and both suffered severe seizure disorders.

What was also common between the two petitioners was that both were diagnosed with the SCN1A gene mutation, more commonly known as Dravet Syndrome. Over the last several years, the court has consistently dismissed petitions where the SCN1A gene mutation, or Dravet Syndrome, was diagnosed.

It is also not the first time that the court has dismissed petitions that claim seizure disorders or where the child has been diagnosed with Dravet Syndrome. A search of the Federal Court of Claims website of petitions that have been adjudicated provides at least a dozen claims of injury. One of the first cases ever to be decided was filed in January 1995, *Gruber v. HHS*. The compensable damage award was entered in August 2005 by Special Master Gary Golkiewicz, awarding actual projected pain and suffering, projected loss of earnings, passed-on reimbursable medical expenses, and compensation for projected vaccine-related medical care. This decision was in 2005 before the pharmaceutical-funded Berkovic study was released.

In another petition filed June 2004, *Stone v. HHS*, Special Master Golkiewicz ruled in May 2011 against the petitioner and dismissed her claim. Upon review, the Federal Court of Claims affirmed the special master's decision. The petitioner appealed the decision up to the Federal Circuit Court of Appeals. In April 2012, the court affirmed the decisions of the Federal Court of Claims and special master, dismissing the petition.

In March 2007 a petition, *Hammitt v. HHS*, was filed with the program claiming that the DTaP vaccination caused the girl to experience a fever, which caused her to experience a prolonged seizure, which damaged her brain, lowering her seizure threshold and therefore facilitating further seizures.[9] The respondent, in filing her Rule 4(c) report,[10] cited medical expert opinions of neurologist Dr. Max Wiznitzer and neurologist and geneticist Dr. Gerald Raymond, both asserting that the young girl's SCN1A gene mutation, not the DTaP vaccination, caused her medical condition.[11] In Special Master Gary Golkiewicz's final decision in March 2011, he noted that the petitioner failed to establish a *prima facie* case, and that even if the petitioner had established a *prima facie* case, the respondent proved by a preponderance of evidence that the SCN1A gene mutation was the sole cause of the young girl's medical condition.

In January 2007 another petition was filed, *Snyder v. HHS*, claiming that the child suffered from epilepsy and seizure disorder as a direct result of the DTaP vaccination. Special Master Christian Moran received the respondent's rule 4(c) report, asserting that it was the child's genetic mutation, the SCN1A gene mutation, that caused his epilepsy and seizure disorder. A hearing was conducted with Dr. Gerald Raymond and Dr. Max Wiznitzer, and both testified that the genetic mutation was the sole cause of the petitioner's epilepsy.[12] In May 2011, Moran issued his decision to deny compensation.

The case of *Snyder v. HHS* illustrates why the program is such a cruel and harsh method to determine compensation for an injured child. In November 2011, upon review in the court of Federal Claims, Judge Susan Braden issued an Opinion and Final Order reversing the special master's dismissal, remanding the petition back to a special master for an award of compensation, reasonable attorney fees, and other costs.[13] In an extremely rare victory for a child suffering from the vaccine injuries of seizure disorder and epilepsy from the administration of the DTaP vaccine, Special Master Christian Moran then filed a decision awarding damages in January 2013.

The damage award was large and will provide financial compensation for future medical care, compensation for lost future earnings, and an annuity to provide steady future income to meet those medical expenses. The government appealed the decision for compensation to the Federal Circuit Court of Appeals. On January 28, 2014, the three-judge panel of the Federal Circuit found in favor of the HHS Secretary, therefore reversing the court of Federal Claims decision and directing the court to reinstate the special master's original decision denying compensation. The special master decision awarding compensation therefore was vacated. The child is still severely injured and is in need of constant and costly medical care. But who pays for that care when the NVICP has turned into an adversarial system, more concerned about policy decisions than of what Congress intended the program to be—fair, quick, and generous to those who suffered vaccine-related injuries or death.

A similar petition and its course of action would follow in the matter of *Harris v. HHS*, filed in January 2007. This child would also receive a decision denying compensation in May of 2011. Special Master Christian Moran, in his decision, stated that the child's epilepsy and seizure disorder was caused by a genetic mutation, the SCN1A mutation, and not by the vaccine. Testifying once again for the respondent were doctors Gerald Raymond and Max Wiznitzer. Upon review, in the Federal Court of Claims, Judge Braden once again reversed Special Master Christian Moran's ruling to dismiss compensation and remanded the petition back to the special master to award compensation. Like the Snyder case before, Harris would receive a compensation award in January 2013 to cover lost future earnings, pain and suffering, and future lifecare expenses in the form of an annuity. And regrettably, much like the Snyder case before, the respondent appealed the compensation award to the Federal Circuit Court of Appeals. On January 28, 2014, the three-judge panel once again found in favor of the HHS Secretary. They reversed the Court of Federal Claims' decision and directed the court to reinstate the special master's decision denying compensation.

There is a dark and ugly pattern emerging from the court's handling of petitions claiming seizure disorder and epilepsy injuries as a result of the DTaP vaccination. If the petitioner submits a claim of seizures and other injuries from the DTaP vaccine, the respondent's position is to automatically claim that the child has the SCN1A gene mutation or Dravet Syndrome; thus their position is to deny compensation by claiming that the gene mutation caused the seizures, and not the vaccine.

In *Deribeaux v. HHS*, an interesting twist developed. The original petition filed in March 2005 claiming seizure disorder and epilepsy would lead to a December 2007 ruling of entitlement decision by Special Master Laura Millman to compensate for damages.[14] The child was diagnosed with atypical Kawasaki disease.[15] There was no mention of SCN1A genetic mutation or Dravet Syndrome. After Special Master Millman's ruling of entitlement decision, the petition would enter the damages phase, where both parties would try to determine future medical needs for the child. During this damages phase, petitioners discovered for the first time in submitted documentation from her treating doctors that the young girl's neurological symptoms could be attributed to Dravet Syndrome or SCN1A gene mutation. The respondent moved to reopen the issue of entitlement. Chief Special Master Gary Golkiewicz transferred the case to Special Master Dee Lord. One has to wonder why the Chief Special Master reassigned the case. Could it be because the original special master would not vacate her decision to compensate?

Once again the respondent called in Dr. Gerald Raymond to assert that the Dravet Syndrome, or SCN1A gene mutation, was the cause of the young girl's seizures and epilepsy episodes.

So on December 9, 2011, Special Master Lord issued her decision to dismiss the petition on the grounds that the respondent had proved by a preponderance of evidence that a factor unrelated to the vaccine, namely the child's genetic mutation, caused her injuries. In June 2012, the petitioner filed motion for review and in the court of Federal Claims, Judge George Miller issued an opinion and order affirming the special master decision to deny compensation. So now we have a unique case where a special master's decision to award compensation was held up in the damages phase. An order was entered to reopen the entitlement decision, and it was reassigned to a different special master, to issue a decision to dismiss. The petitioner appealed Judge Miller's opinion and the Federal Circuit Court of Appeals decision on June 7, 2013, affirms Special Master Lord's decision to dismiss the petition.

Another development that is disturbing from the case decisions, opinions and orders from the Federal Court of Claims, and decisions from the Federal Circuit Court of Appeals is the following: It appears that the Federal Circuit is basically allowing special masters to compel petitioners to test for the gene mutation SCN1A or Dravet Syndrome because of the late development of determination or disclosure in *Deribeaux v. HHS*. Will this open the door for a much broader interpretation down the road requiring genetic testing for more vaccine-related injuries? This is a concern that we all should share. For to allow the courts to require or compel genetic testing of petitioners who file claims with vaccine injury or seizure disorders or other injuries would mean that the court and our government are moving in a direction in which medical conditions that arise from the administration of vaccines are more about genetic conditions than vaccine injury.

It is also important to note that while I introduced several petitions and went into a detailed discussion of each, there was also a trend developing of denying compensation for any petition once the respondent introduced the Berkovic or McIntosh study and brought in their reliable medical experts of Dr. Gerald Raymond and Dr. Max Wiznitzer.

Another emerging concern that I have noticed while examining several petitions and case decisions regarding Dravet Syndrome is that the respondent has taken the position that if the petitioner has been tested and confirmed with Dravet Syndrome, their petition will be automatically dismissed. It is starting to look like what happened back prior to 1995 for those injured children who filed petitions claiming they suffered from seizure disorders after receiving the DPT vaccine. In 1995, the HHS Secretary removed Residual Seizure Disorder (RSD) from the Vaccine Injury Table (VIT), thus dismissing hundreds of petitions that were pending and preventing future petitions from compensation. And it appears that the respondent is now doing this again by denying compensation for petitioners who suffer from vaccine-related injuries such as seizures and epilepsy after receiving the DTaP vaccination.

By removing Residual Seizure Disorder and now setting precedent in the court system of denying compensation for seizures and epilepsy, the government has severely limited those who have been injured by vaccines. Is it a coincidence that the two leading studies used by our government to deny compensation originated in Australia? Combined with a recent article published in Australia, promoting the idea to bring back the DPT whole cell vaccination,[16] it does appear that plans are being made to bring back the unsafe DPT vaccine. This vaccine, as effective as it was against whooping cough, also killed many children and injured thousands. It was parents of injured children from the DPT back in the early 1980s that lobbied Congress extensively to create the National Vaccine Injury Compensation Program. So why would we want to return to that horrible vaccine that maimed and injured so many?

Our government and medical community along with the CDC have been campaigning over the last several years, claiming the whooping cough outbreaks are the fault of parents not vaccinating their children. In fact, it is because of the waning efficacy or inability to combat the pertussis bacteria of the DTaP vaccine. According to an article in *Scientific American* from May 2013, research scientists really do not know why the DTaP vaccine is only approximately 25 percent as effective as the DPT.[17]

Health officials are now blaming the children and their genetic makeup. It has not been proven, and it is quite possible that the over-vaccination and other environmental assaults are causing mutations in our genes. They allege that if a child has some underlying medical condition or genetic disposition, such as mitochondrial dysfunction or an SCN1A gene mutation, then that is the root of the problem, but certainly not the vaccine.

More credible research is required. It is the continued dialogue that it is the child's fault, that it is not the vaccine's fault, because the vaccine is safe, is such a ridiculous argument. But for many, they are buying it without any questions or challenging the conclusions.

So the groundwork has been laid to relicense some form of the DPT vaccine without any concern about all the future injured children and those who will die from it. They have already closed the barn door and thrown away the keys on compensation in the NVICP for seizure disorders.

Are we heading in a direction where the medical community, the vaccine manufacturers, and our government will dictate that most or all vaccine-related brain injuries are the result of genetic makeup instead of being the result of severe reactions to vaccination?

Are the courts, the DOJ attorneys, and the HHS Secretary revising history, or are they trying to make so many children relive it?

Chapter 12

Intimidation

The Merriam-Webster dictionary defines intimidation as: to make timid or fearful: frighten; especially: to compel or deter by or as if by threats; try to intimidate a witness.

For families and parents of children who have filed petitions in the NVICP, the word *intimidation* will describe the actions of DOJ attorneys and their conduct toward them and their medical experts during hearings and also during negotiations after damages have been awarded.

Intimidation is also the word to describe the pro-Pharma media and Internet bloggers who write articles trying to defame the reputations of families who have won compensation in the NVICP. Certain medical practitioners who are in a state of denial regarding vaccine injury will constantly promote that it was the fault of the children, their genetics, or other factors that caused severe reactions to vaccines.

And there are the more famous intimidation attempts by the medical community and media against scientists and researchers who question the safety of certain vaccinations. There are stories of university researchers or legal scholars who question vaccination policies, later to learn their employment, research grants, and funding are threatened.

I have written previously about one mother who advocates for safer vaccines because she claims it was a vaccine that killed her daughter. She spoke about her daughter and claims in front of a national audience with a TV talk show host. Within hours of the airing of the program, Internet bloggers were out, posting false articles about her character, misquoting the facts of the specific case, all done to intimidate her and those in the future who will face the same unfortunate tragedy. There is no argument for a civil discussion of the facts, however, when it is apparent that the agenda is to manipulate the facts, to defame the character, and to intimidate others, perhaps so that those in the media and individuals from both sides of the issue refrain from the discussion.

These intimidation attempts are not scattered or random. There is a clear agenda by pharmaceutical companies using nonprofit organizations, like-minded health media columnists, reporters, and bloggers, plus certain medical practitioners as their proxies to deliver a message to family members and parents who have filed petitions in the NVICP, and especially to deliver hostile treatment toward those who have won compensation. Some of the intimidation is straightforward, but other attempts are accomplished in subtle terms. Some families live in fear of their government, such as unwarranted IRS audits, or DOJ attorneys questioning the compensation awards and the daily operations of the trust accounts.

Prior to the Omnibus Autism Proceedings, many medical experts who testifed for a petitioner were treated with respect during a hearing and when being cross-examined by DOJ attorneys. However, during the OAP that was not true. DOJ attorneys would hold their own medical experts in high regard, a sense of reverence. And when cross-examining experts, the attorneys threw all politeness and respect out the window. Congress intended the entire process of the NVICP to be less adversarial, and that meant including how medical experts were treated as well as the petitioners and their families. That common courtesy all changed once the OAP conducted its first hearings in June 2007, and it continues today.

I conducted many interviews with families who won compensation and yet refused to go on the record to discuss their experiences, nor would they talk about their journey with the NVICP with business associates or neighbors. They felt isolated, even when the medical science shows that their child suffered severe injuries and will have to live with a medical condition that requires constant medical attention and care for the rest of their lives. Surprisingly, some of them are prominent members of their community, but their friends and neighbors are informed.

The following story is about how government attorneys and their representatives, who at the petitioner's weakest moment try to intimidate and harass to accomplish a significant concession.

Lorrin Kain

Lorrin was born April 1994 to parents Tom and Karen Kain. She entered this world with a bright smile and a twinkle in her eye. And that would soon change.

During Lorrin's well-baby checkup six weeks later, the pediatrician administered the DPT vaccine. Lorrin had a severe adverse reaction to this vaccine and it was later determined that this vaccine was part of a "hot lot" batch. Lorrin suffered acute encephalopathy, seizures, blindness, and partial hearing loss.

As new parents, Tom and Karen struggled to determine why this happened and more importantly what could be done to help Lorrin and her recovery. Lorrin would constantly suffer from seizures. Her doctors continued to administer one medication after another, trying to control her seizure episodes. However, these medications did not work and it took several months to wean Lorrin off one before administering another.

Karen listened to the doctors, but they couldn't answer her questions about how this happened to Lorrin. In 1994 the Internet was in its infancy; however, Karen became a determined mother researching all possibilities including vaccine injury. Lorrin's doctors continued to deny a correlation between her medical condition and the vaccine. It wasn't until the discovery that that specific vaccine administered to Lorrin was part of a hot lot as declared by the vaccine manufacturer that it was taken seriously.

When a doctor or clinic or hospital receives an order of a specific vaccine, generally in boxes of twenty, those vaccines in that box would be from different manufacturing lots, therefore ensuring that no two vaccines received are from the same manufacturing lot or batch, and thus a doctor or hospital would not witness multiple injuries if indeed the entire lot was damaged. But it also makes it extremely difficult to trace or to assess. The specific vaccine that Lorrin received was from a known hot lot. Did the FDA or the CDC trace the remaining vaccines of that lot and notify the doctors, the clinics, or hospitals and withdraw that vaccine?

What should be concerning to the American people is that neither the FDA nor the CDC required the vaccine manufacturers to disclose the number of vaccines in that production lot. This number is kept secret and so the number of suspected injuries from the specific lot of vaccines cannot be determined.

During Karen's research on vaccine injury she became aware of the National Vaccine Injury Compensation Program and wondered if she would be eligible to file a claim or a petition with the program to seek compensation for vaccine-related injuries to her daughter. Along the way, as Karen was starting to inquire about the process of filing a petition, an attorney was recommended to her.

Andrew Dodd had an extensive resume of filing petitions on the behalf of vaccine-injured children. On March 6, 1995, Karen filed a petition with the NVICP. Special Master E. LaVon French was assigned to preside over the petition process. Karen worked extensively around the clock with her attorney to obtain and gather all the necessary medical records, documentation, and other materials that would be necessary to successfully prosecute her petition.

Within ninety days of filing her petition, the respondent filed a report with the court agreeing with the vaccine injury and Lorrin's medical condition. Special Master French then directed a court-appointed life care planner to interview the family and to file a report with the court as to the anticipated future medical expenses for Lorrin. It appeared that the petition of *Lorrin Kain v. HHS* was proceeding favorably. However, the process would slowly grind to a halt and become adversarial during the negotiations of the life care plan to be established for Lorrin.

The initial meeting to discuss the future and ongoing medical care for Lorrin began in Lorrin's attorney's office. Special Master French, along with the government's attorney, a nurse, and a pediatrician would review the life care plan.

At the very beginning of the negotiations the respondent recommended that Lorrin be placed in a home, away from her parents. Karen refused, and the negotiations turned from a civil discussion and escalated to an adversarial debate over the medical care needed for Lorrin.

With over eighty specific items to be discussed, this process would take three days, and according to Karen it would become one of the worst periods in her life. According to her the environment in the room was toxic. The government's nurse made readily apparent to Karen that Lorrin's life really meant nothing and that Karen was of no importance either. As they started to discuss the list of specific items, the government's nurse and her constant insults toward Karen became so offensive that the special master threatened to kick her out of the room.

Both the respondent's nurse and the government attorney were playing off each other and were constantly insulting Karen and becoming extremely argumentative on every item in the specific list. The intimidation continued as a discussion lasted over twenty minutes regarding the cost of baby wipes and whether to use brand-name or a generic brand. The nurse continued her intimidation tactics by questioning Karen on why she changed Lorrin so many times each day. As the discussions over the list drew to a close on the third day, most of the items outlined by the life care planner were eliminated from the list. Thus the government's attorney and the nurse who had never interviewed or spent time with Lorrin prior to this three-day meeting achieved what they sought in the beginning. And that is to intimidate, insult, and pound the petitioners so as to make them accept whatever the respondent decided was in the best interests of the child.

The respondent, however, did meet Lorrin, but with dubious motivation. Instead of inquiring how was she doing, they inspected Lorrin for bruising and took off her diaper to look for bedsores. What they were doing was trying to find evidence that Karen or Tom were bad parents and neglecting their daughter, trying to find another escape clause out of compensating for a vaccine injury.

As the process of negotiating a life care plan became confrontational, intimidating, Karen's biggest fear was starting to play out. It was no secret that in Lorrin's medical records, her doctors were concerned that Lorrin could pass soon due to her seizure episodes. And Karen thought that the government would now slowplay or delay in their decisions regarding compensation amounts, in hopes that Lorrin would pass, thus eliminating a costly compensation damage award.

This delaying tactic is nothing new and has been considered a practice by the respondent with many petitioners who are eligible to receive monetary damages. This would, however, all come to a close on February 5, 1998, in Special Master French's decision to award damages and agree upon the exact amount.

Karen was extremely impressed with Mr. Dodd and his handling of Lorrin's petition through the adversarial and intimidating process of negotiating a life care plan. However, according to Karen, Mr. Dodd failed in one area. It is the responsibility of the petitioner's attorney to contact each state's Medicaid/Medicare agency to inquire about any medical care or service provided to the petitioner. This is done prior to the final decision and agreement of compensation. The vaccine injury trust fund would reimburse that state's Medicaid/Medicare agency for any services provided. This was not done. Because of this, California DHS filed a lien against Lorrin's estate immediately after it received compensation.

After a lengthy court battle and an appeal, the state of California prevailed and Lorrin's estate would have to reimburse all medical expenses provided to Lorrin by the state of California.

After all this, dealing with the unknown cause of Lorrin's medical condition, searching for the best medical care for Lorrin, the denial of her doctors of a vaccine-related injury, the legal process of filing a petition, listening to the respondent's attorney and nurse trying their best to humiliate and intimidate, and to ultimately win compensation for her daughter, Karen was now in a position to dedicate all of her efforts and resources to providing her daughter with the best chance, an opportunity to fully live the life that she deserved.

Lorrin would continue to defy all medical doctors, and she taught her mother and others to be in the moment, to get up and take on the day. Lorrin would pass in December 2009 at the age of fifteen. She was a tremendous source of inspiration for her mother, and now Karen is a tremendous source of inspiration to many others. Karen has written a book about her daughter Lorrin and the life that she led, *A Unique Life Fully Lived: A Personal Journey of Love, Hope, And Courage.*

Chapter 13

Moving Too Fast?

Over the past couple of years in the NVICP, there has been a disturbing trend regarding the adjudicating of human papillomavirus (HPV) petitions in a timely matter. Almost all of us know about the controversial vaccine licensed in the United States and around the world to "prevent" cervical cancer; Gardasil by Merck and Cervarix by GlaxoSmithKline are licensed to help protect against HPV infection. Gardasil was initially approved in June 2006 in the United States. Cervarix, in October 2009, was licensed in the United States for females only.

As of March 2014, there have been 224 HPV-related petitions filed in the NVICP, with the court awarding compensation in sixty-nine claims and dismissing sixty-nine claims. The remaining 86 petitions are pending adjudication. A disturbing trend is the rate of how fast the petitions are being processed. Since HPV vaccines are an extremely new vaccine in the market, the actual research on adverse reactions and ongoing safety studies has not been developed sufficiently.

The current Vaccine Injury Table for HPV vaccines has been considered by attorneys who represent HPV-injured petitioners and other advocates as extremely narrow and not as thorough as other vaccines when first accepted into the program.[1] One attorney who represents several petitioners mentioned to me that "because HPV vaccine injury or death is often autoimmune in nature, and the injury/death is so unique when compared to another HPV petition, it is very bizarre."[2]

After reading case decisions in over 100 HPV adjudications, there are hardly any common similarities.[3] This brings us back to the point of a disturbing trend. These petitions are being adjudicated at an alarming rate for relating to a new vaccine with unique injuries or causation of death. A careful reading shows the special masters are trying to figure out how to handle these cases and make lawful decisions. The comment that has been mentioned by a few medical experts in several of the petitions is that "the science is so new, the research and study to carefully examine all of the conditions is not broad based."[4]

Because the table is so narrowly defined, most of the petitions for HPV vaccine-related injury or death are automatically adjudicated as causation cases.[5] In the program, if the petitioner can show that the injury/death is listed in the table as an on-table injury, the petitioner is eligible for compensation unless the respondent can prove that something other than the vaccine caused the injury/death. However, most of the injuries show medical conditions that are not listed in the table; thus the petitioner must prove causation.

Currently, a petitioner must prove causation by fulfilling the Althen standard. To review, in *Althen v. HHS*, the court determined that in order to prevail in causation, the petitioner must comply with the three-prong test by providing:[6]

1) a medical theory causally connecting the vaccination and the injury (can cause);
2) a logical sequence of cause and effect showing that the vaccination was the reason for the injury (did cause); and
3) showing of a proximate temporal relationship between vaccination and injury.

To show causation, the petitioner is not required to supply epidemiologic or other medical literature supporting the causation.[7] However, if the literature is offered and placed into the record, the special master can use that material in his or her deliberation.[8]

Now, how does this apply to the HPV petitioners who are currently being adjudicated? Let's examine a few of them and see how these standards are being applied to the petition.

* * *

In *Flores v. HHS*,[9] a young girl received two Gardasil vaccinations at the age of fourteen, during the summer of 2008. Within twenty-four hours after receiving the second vaccination, she was rushed to the hospital by ambulance, awoke during the ride and complained of weakness on her entire left side and a shortness of breath. Also, she mentioned that she had a severe headache. Later that day she developed paralysis and loss of sensation. Her mother told the hospital staff that her daughter, the day before, had just received the second Gardasil vaccination.

The hospital performed many tests to determine the cause of her medical condition. In one of the genetic work-up tests, a common genetic abnormality was discovered. Infectious disease tests came back negative. She remained in the hospital as the staff moved away from heart-related causes and was given a working diagnosis of transverse myelitis. Five weeks later, two neurologists who were reviewing her case opined that given this girl's quick onset, absence of inflammatory markers, and a lack of response to anti-inflammatory treatment, they favored a vascular etiology. One neurologist also commented that the HPV vaccination was too close to the symptom onset. The other neurologist noted that he doubted an autoimmune etiology.

She would be transferred to a long-term rehabilitation facility nearly forty days after being rushed to the hospital. During her stay, she remained on a ventilator and her physical abilities did not improve. She also had great difficulty in speaking. She would finally return home six months after her ordeal started. She was confined to a wheelchair and was dependent on a full-time ventilator and care provided to her by her mother and home health nurse. Medical experts reviewing her medical history would later determine that she suffered a spinal cord stroke.

In *Flores v. HHS* filed two years later, the petitioner contended that she suffered a stroke that was "caused in fact" by her second HPV vaccination. The special master assigned to the petition concluded that she failed to demonstrate the vaccine causation of her injury.[10]

A medical expert for the petitioner and the medical experts for the respondent all agreed that a blood clot caused her spinal cord stroke.[11] However, the experts for the respondent contended that the causation of the blood clot was not from the vaccine and that Gardasil has not been associated with blood clots or spinal cord infarction.[12] There is no record of any previous blood clotting or stroke in the girl's medical history. So how did this happen?

The respondent medical experts stated that a gene mutation does not cause blood clotting.[13] The special master concluded that the medical expert for the petitioner failed to establish that the petitioner had a genetic predisposition that made her susceptible to having blood clots. In summary, the medical experts for the respondent were able to provide some limited research that nullified any theories advanced by the medical expert for the petitioner. Thus, the special master's own comment in the decision was "this is not a close case."[14]

According to established case law, that might be the case, that the special master followed Althen and decided that the petitioner failed prongs 1 and 2. However, we need to think about what would happen if there were more credible science or studies that could be advanced for the next petitioner? So what caused this fourteen-year-old girl to have a spinal cord stroke? All we know is that the NVICP decided it was not Gardasil because of two medical experts defending the respondent's position that the vaccine could not have caused the stroke. We know that the girl, now twenty years of age, will be confined to a wheelchair while depending on a ventilator to breathe. With the help of a home health nurse and her mother, maybe, just maybe, she can slowly improve. And no doctor was able to determine what caused the specific blood clot.[15]

* * *

For several petitions, the parties have agreed to settle the case and negotiate on a dollar figure. What the public and the medical community are not informed about are the facts or medical conditions related to the injuries received and subsequent death.

Kristina received two HPV vaccinations in April and June of 2008. Her mother filed a petition with the NVICP claiming that Kristina died as a result of the HPV vaccination.[16] The respondent denied that the HPV vaccine caused Kristina's injuries and death. Nonetheless, both parties agreed to settle this case. The mother of Kristina accepted a compensable damage award of $20,000 that represented compensation for all damages. In petitions regarding vaccine-related death, the damage award can compensate up to a maximum cap of $250,000.

There is little to study after reading the case decision. Petitioner alleged that Kristina developed Weston Hurst disease and/or acute disseminated encephalomyelitis (ADEM), and/or juvenile amyotrophic lateral sclerosis (ALS), and/or chronic, progressive demyelinating encephalitis that led to her death.[17]

What is missing from this case is the fact that no medical experts, testimony, or medical literature has been forwarded. The process involved the petition being filed in February 2011, mountains of medical records and other documents being filed, and both parties negotiating a settlement. No hearings were conducted.

And now, we will not know the true extent of whether the HPV vaccination did, in fact, cause the vaccine-related injuries to Kristina and ultimately led to her death. We have a grieving parent and the general public wanting answers and the government, the respondent, having a talking point that the HPV vaccine did not cause this death.

* * *

In another HPV vaccine-related death petition filed in 2010, Teri claimed that the two HPV vaccinations that her daughter received in October 2007 and on March 31, 2008, caused her death just a week after receiving the second HPV vaccination.[18]

After the initial filing, the petitioner filed additional medical records and other documents. It would be nearly eighteen months later that medical expert reports filed on the behalf of the petitioner would be placed into the record. The special master conducted a hearing nearly three and a half years after the filing and issued a decision denying compensation. In the decision, a one-page decision, the special master ruled that the petitioner did not establish by a preponderance of the evidence the first two prongs of Althen.

The troubling part of this decision was that it was only one page in length. The special master went to considerable effort to refrain from publishing any more details than what would fit on one page. So why did the petitioner fail the first two prongs of the Althen standard? We will never know.

There have been several instances where the Federal Court of Claims judges scolded special masters for not writing a descriptive decision. This is necessary in the evaluation process in case the petitioner or respondent filed a motion for review. With a lack of information and the proceedings of the hearing, you must ask the question, is the special master or government hiding something that they do not want to be made public? Independent research to develop a medical outcome of this tragedy and knowledge about what medical conditions can result from the HPV vaccine are squelched.

The court has adjudicated HPV cases for the last three years. We know very little about the medical history and whether there are causation factors that will not be made public, due to the overeagerness of the court and our government to quickly deal with petitions before independent science and research catches up, or just agreeing to settle so that the details of the specific case are not made public.

Chapter 14

Dare to Reform?

If there is an area that the vaccine attorneys representing petitioners, DOJ attorneys who represent the HHS Secretary as the respondent, parent advocates, and legal scholars can all agree upon, it is the idea the National Vaccine Injury Compensation Program as originally passed in 1986 is not the same program today. Not even close.

But what can we do about it? Even though each of the groups mentioned above has different ideas on what happened to the program, all are in agreement that if the program is to continue, it must be reformed. And most of the reform measures that have been proposed need Congressional input.

So let's take a look at some of the more discussed measures and analyze how they will improve the program. We also must be careful to point out that proponents of reform measures in the past might not be so eager to promote those very same reform measures now. Meaning, have we passed over the point of no return?

The following represent some of the more popular or debated reform measures that Congress and the court should entertain.

1. Expand the Statute of Limitations.

One of the most discussed reform measures to the program would be to expand the limiting statute of limitations. Currently, the petitioner has three years from the date of first onset of illness or symptoms of a suspected vaccine injury to file.[1] In the case of death, the representative of the estate has two years to file from the date of the death and within four years of the first symptom that leads to the death of the individual.[2]

The original act mandated that the purpose of the program was to be fair, quick, and generous to those who suffered vaccine-related injury or death. By no means could Congress envision all the new vaccines to be added to the table and the subsequent vaccine-related injuries that can take months if not years to manifest themselves.

By expanding the statute of limitations to six years or even ten years, it would restore the meaning of "generous" to the program. The HHS Secretary's own Advisory Commission on Childhood Vaccines (ACCV) has recommended on several occasions to expand the statute of limitations to six years. There have been previous attempts by Congress, most notably by Congressman Dan Burton of Indiana, to introduce legislation to increase the period from three years to six years. Several attorneys who practice within the program have even suggested expanding the statute out to the age of eighteen for children.

However, the recommendations from the ACCV and attempts to expand by legislation have gone nowhere. If the statute is ever expanded, it has been highly suggested to allow the special masters to have the option of reconsidering old cases dismissed for late filing that would have met the new statute of limitation's deadline.[3]

2. Revise the Vaccine Injury Table to reflect the intentions of Congress.

As Barbara Loe Fisher pointed out in her testimony in front of the House Subcommittee on September 28, 1999:

"The principal reason why the Vaccine Injury Compensation Program has become highly adversarial and is turning away three out of four claimants is that the Department of Health and Human Services (DHHS), with the assistance of the Department of Justice (DOJ), has wielded its discretionary authority to all but eliminate a just list of compensable events in the Vaccine Injury Table, thereby destroying the guiding tenet of presumption. This action by DHHS constitutes the most egregious violation of the spirit and intent of the law and, in effect, is a fatal compromise of its integrity."

One prominent attorney in the NVICP is Cliff Shoemaker. In his testimony to Congress, he suggested a complete roll-back of the Vaccine Injury Table amendments: "reinstate the table of injuries originally created by Congress and remove the Secretary's power to change the table in such a way as to make it more difficult to receive compensation."[4]

It has been suggested by several individuals to remove the HHS Secretary out of the equation for table determination and to place that responsibility with the ACCV or another committee with a cross-section of representation from petitioners, attorneys, and medical professionals.

The changes to the VIT in 1995 and the follow-up in 1997 led to the changing of the program from being a "generous, fair, and quick" process to a highly adversarial, litigious, and lengthy process. The HHS Secretary at the time, Donna Shalala, based her decision on the report from the Institute of Medicine, which is highly questionable. In his critique of the action of the secretary, Peter Meyers wrote the following: "Several persons who submitted comments to the Secretary on the proposed new table pointed out that the Secretary had not considered the results of several large databases on vaccine injuries, and urged the Secretary to wait for more definitive information before modifying the table."[5]

The Secretary responded that it was unnecessary for the information it relied upon to be "definite and conclusive before any changes are made." Several persons also submitted comments indicating that the 1995 rule change would substantially change the nature of the NVICP, but the secretary responded that "the benefits of the proposed regulations outweigh the possibility of more protracted and complex hearings."[6]

The question that needs to be asked based on the comments by the secretary is this: What benefit will be achieved and who is going to benefit from the proposed changes?[7]

According to former Chief Special Master Gary Golkiewicz, commenting about the 1995 rule change in his decision of *Stevens v. HHS*, "with the changes to the table and the subsequent addition of many new vaccines without any new table injuries, the focus of vaccine case adjudication is now dramatically different. In the beginning, 90 percent of all petitions were on-table injuries. Now, 90 percent of all petitions are now causation-in-fact cases."[8]

3. Increase the Death Benefit.

Congress outlined in statute that the compensable award for vaccine-related death would be capped at $250,000.[9] This award also had an inflation index attached. That index was removed a couple of years later as part of a Congressional Omnibus Reconciliation Bill. There have been multiple attempts by Congressman Dan Burton of Indiana to increase the monetary cap and also restore the inflation index. Also, the ACCV has proposed recently to increase the cap to be adjusted for inflation in their recommendation to the HHS Secretary.[10]

Everyone knows that $250,000 in 1986 dollars does not equate to the same amount in today's currency. Applying the US Department of Labor Statistics Inflation calculator, the $250,000 would be equal in 2014 dollars to approximately $530,000.

Another way to view the inadequacy of the death benefit is to compare it against other successful compensation programs. Using the September 11th Victim Compensation Fund, a petitioner would file a claim for compensation as a result of the terrorist attacks for the loss of a family member or injuries sustained at the World Trade Center, the Pentagon, or at Shanksville, Pennsylvania.[11] There was no artificial cap for a damage award. The objectives of the Fund would be to compensate the eligible parties generously, promptly, and fairly. This is similar language to the NVICP, describing the objectives. But that is where the similarity stops. The September 11th Fund awarded compensation for 5,560 claims.[12] The average award involving the death of a claimant was $2,082,035,[13] over eight times the cap in the NVICP.[14]

Congress needs to reexamine the death benefit statute and increase the dollar amount to levels found in similar compensation programs such as the September 11th Fund.

4. Publish the attorney fees and medical expert fees and costs incurred by the respondent.

The Vaccine Act allows for decisions regarding the attorney fees and medical expert costs that represent the petitioner to be published. This allows the general public the ability to review these costs and also provide comment to the court regarding the fees. What is missing is how much the respondent charges for attorney fees (DOJ) or the medical expert costs for both the internal review (medical doctors on staff with the DVIC) and those experts retained by the DOJ or HHS to defend their position. There have been several attempts or recommendations to ask DOJ and HHS to publish these costs, all to be denied on the grounds of "it would divulge their legal strategy." Sounds nice, but it is just a bunch of bull. FOIA requests by this author and others to release fees and costs for specific cases have been ignored based upon "privileged information." This is not someone asking the White House to provide transcripts of certain meetings with the president or vice president with industry leaders. Matter of fact, since the taxpayers pay for most of the budgets of DOJ and HHS, what we do not know is how much of the Vaccine Injury Trust Fund is being used to pay for these expenses and how much is being paid via our taxes.

Petitioner attorney fees and medical expert expenses are reviewed by the respondent and the special master. This process happens in all court systems. But what does not happen is the petitioner having the same opportunity to review respondent expenses. It is a one-way street. More transparency of transactions and costs within the NVICP will help create an equitable program.

5. Reexamine the redaction process to help protect the identity and medical history of the vaccine injured or those who have died as a result of a vaccine.

There is no statute, rule, or decision to support a petitioner's request for total anonymity.[15] Under the E-Government Act, which applies to the Office of Special Masters (OSM), a unit of the US Court of Federal Claims, the courts have adopted rules governing redaction of private information.[16]

6. More transparency regarding the posting of adjudications on HRSA's website, including how many petitions are filed each year by vaccine injury or vaccine type.

Not all final decisions are posted on the court's website. Therefore, the public does not know the extent of how many petitions are actually compensated or dismissed by each vaccine type. Currently, there are some statistics that are posted on the HRSA website. But they are not final and are always subject to adjustment without acknowledgment of the cause. This author has been a keen student of the monthly statistics published by HRSA. Yet for reasons unknown, a statistic will be changed without acknowledgment. And some of the figures could be statistics from several months ago or even years ago.

The current statistics are maintained by a third party instead of being maintained and audited for accuracy by HRSA. DVIC created a new report that is posted on the HRSA statistics website. It publicizes the number of vaccines distributed each year since 2006 compared to the number of petitions adjudicated.[17] Clearly the message by DVIC is to illustrate to the public that petitions claiming injury are very small compared to the number of vaccines distributed. Let alone that distributed is a large number compared to the actual number of vaccines administered. And why start with the year 2006? DVIC has the data, why don't they post by each fiscal year?

7. Congress directs the HHS Secretary to conduct a continuous Public Awareness Campaign on the NVICP as mandated by statute.

By continuing to rely on educating the general public via VIS statements, the actions of the HHS Secretary will ensure more people will not know their rights or options to file a petition within the NVICP. The continued practice of medical practitioners denying that medical conditions or diseases might be related to a vaccination is misleading the public. With more vaccines being introduced, vaccine-related injury or death is rare, but it does exist. And with the current trend of vaccine-related injuries being autoimmune in nature, most injuries are not easily diagnosed or do not manifest themselves quickly.

The ACCV committee proposed a public awareness campaign in 2009 and 2010 and solicited Banyan Communications to develop the campaign. The proposed campaign was suddenly stopped in 2010. Maybe there was pushback from the medical community and the pharmaceutical industry about their worries that a large number of people would file petitions in the NVICP or the general public would start to question the "actual" safety of vaccinations.

8. Require the GAO and the HHS Inspector General to conduct reviews and audits of the program and the Vaccine Injury Trust Fund on a regular basis.

Most people have been told that for every vaccine sold in the United States, a tax of $0.75 will be levied and the proceeds will be placed in trust to the Vaccine Injury Trust Fund. As I disclosed in earlier chapters, that is not the case. According to an IRS statute and also from presentations made in the ACCV committee, 25 percent of the revenue actually is placed into the General Fund of the US Treasury and is never placed into the Trust Fund. For every $0.75 vaccine levy, $0.19 will be sent directly to the federal government to be used for fighting a foreign war, funding for the arts, paying for new highway interstate road construction, or other funding needs of the government, but not for those who are vaccine injured or who have died. Only $0.56 is being placed into the Trust Fund instead of the $0.75 that is commonly reported. Or is it? We do not know if more money is being siphoned off to fund other budgets, or if the process of our federal government confiscating 25 percent of the income has been halted and the entire $0.75 is going directly to the Trust Fund.

And we do not know how many vaccines are actually sold each year. On the HRSA website, a report designed by the Division of Vaccine Injury Compensation shows an aggregate number of vaccines distributed. But no one can determine how many were sold each year. And what is the difference between distributed versus sold?

According to balance sheets and income statements published on a monthly basis and posted on the US Treasury's website, the Trust Fund has been growing every year, and is currently approaching $3.5 billion. Each year, Congress appropriates money out of the Trust

Fund and forwards it to the three agencies that have direct administrative duties of the program: the Department of Justice, the Federal Court of Claims, and Health Resources and Services Administration (HRSA), a unit of HHS. The Department of Justice provides attorneys to represent the respondent, the HHS Secretary, in all petitions. Their fees and costs are reimbursed by the Trust Fund yet they are not published, and are not subject to review by petitioner attorneys. DOJ attorneys hide behind the "privileged material and would divulge their legal strategy" as the reason for not posting their fees and costs, contrary to the petitioner's attorneys. The Federal Court of Claims is reimbursed for all salaries, fees, and costs for the special masters and associated staff, office rents, and other costs. HRSA receives the largest reimbursement of fees and costs from the Trust Fund mainly due to the agency's duty to fund the compensation to the petitioners for awards received, including an annuity program, plus petitioner's attorney fees and their medical experts costs. The public is made aware of all compensable awards and legal and medical expert fees. HRSA also receives reimbursement for administering the program. However, this is where an audit needs to be conducted. The amount of money paid to HRSA each year up and beyond the damage awards is growing.

There is considerable criticism that the government agencies that receive reimbursement from the Trust Fund are actually balancing their budget shortfalls or circumventing their budgets from the federal sequester. This author has forwarded FOIA requests to HRSA, DOJ, and the courts asking for a detailed report of the amount of money requested from the Trust Fund that pays for administration duties in the program. Those FOIA requests have been ignored.

There is also considerable speculation that certain expenses are being paid by the Trust Fund that would be a clear violation of Federal law and the Vaccine Act. These expenses consist of vaccine research done by the Institute of Medicine and funded by HRSA. A few highly placed officials and committee members suspected monies from the Trust Fund were actually used, disguised as appropriations to HRSA. FOIA's submitted to HRSA asking for all documents, expense reports, funding approval, and other associated materials have been ignored.

9. Create a review board to analyze all petitions that take over three years to adjudicate.

Are there trends or procedures that are noticeable or can be streamlined to help future petitions on the front end? Another idea is to recruit retired special masters or judges to become part of the review board or advisory committee to the court.

10. Expedite the interim fee applications from petitioner attorneys, especially the medical experts.

The courts hold a hammer over the petitioner, especially their attorneys and medical experts, regarding how fast to reimburse fees and costs. It is becoming difficult to retain a medical expert, especially as new vaccines are being introduced, and a new era of autoimmune disorders and diseases are being associated with vaccination.

The court and DOJ have a long history of intimidation of medical experts who testify on the behalf of petitioners. The medical experts charge a fee for their specialized training, education, and research experience. If they are subject to having the reimbursement delayed or their invoices challenged unnecessarily, many will not return. And that just might be the game plan for the respondent.

11. Requiring special masters to publish, in all decisions, including stipulations, proffers, and rulings for entitlement, the vaccine(s) and the nature of the injury or disease.

A major tenet of the Vaccine Act is "to advance the public heath through the collection and dissemination of information about vaccines, including adverse events potentially related to vaccine administrations, and through promoting the development of safer vaccines."[18]

In many stipulated decisions (agreement to settle between both parties), the use of vague language, such as "suffered a neurological injury, and that this condition was either caused-in-fact or significantly aggravated by the influenza vaccination," does nothing to "advance the public health." The respondent does assert that they deny that the petitioner's vaccinations caused her injuries. Then the special master finds the stipulation reasonable and adopts it as the decision of the court and awards compensation.[19]

So what has the public learned from this? Nothing other than that a compensable damage award was decided. The public might want to think that an influenza vaccination caused a neurological injury; however, with some clever legal language, our government is in a position to "legally" state that there was no injury, but we agreed to settle. Just write the petitioner a check and go away.

Transparency has a way of cutting through all fog created by the legal maneuvering, applying a little disinfectant, to allow the general public a better view of injuries occurred by vaccination.

12. For vaccines that are not listed in the NVICP, a modification to the VIS published by the CDC, to state that the (specific) vaccine is not included in the NVICP.

As required by statute, all vaccines licensed and administered for the general public have a corresponding Vaccine Information Statement listing general information about the vaccine such as who should receive it, who should not get the vaccine or should wait, what the risks are, and what to do if there is a serious reaction, including reporting all serious reactions to VAERS. For those vaccines that are listed in the NVICP, there is information included in the VIS regarding the program and how to learn about the program. What is not included for those vaccinations that are not listed in the NVICP is information instructing the person that the NVICP does not cover any vaccine-related injuries or death as a result of that specific vaccine. This has led to confusion with several individuals who have been injured, filed a petition, and then several months later when the decision is handed down, these people learn that the petition has been dismissed because the court lacks subject-matter jurisdiction in adjudicating the petition.[20]

The general public and the court would be better served if VIS statements for vaccines not covered by the NVICP have a notation stating that fact.

13. Allowing parents or spouse to file claims in the NVICP.

We need to continue the work of the ACCV workgroup's 2007 recommendation of amending the act to allow parents or spouses to file petitions in the NVICP seeking compensation for damages, including claims for loss of consortium, society companionship or services, loss of earnings while providing medical care for their family member, or other expenses and emotional distress.[21]

There are many cases of which the petitioner did receive compensation for their injury. However, the family members suffered as well. For several, the loss of a home due to foreclosure because of a working spouse or parent having to quit the workforce to help provide medical care for their family member, or the pain and suffering endured by the rest of the family while waiting five, six, or even ten years until the petition was adjudicated.

Those expenses are more difficult to determine, but the pain and suffering by the family, the sacrificing by the parent or spouse, is just as real.

Porter Bridges

Having your four-month-old child rushed to the ER is one of the scariest events for parents. Not knowing what is happening, not knowing what the outcome will be, and not knowing what caused Porter to have seizures and stop breathing, Dr. Sarah Bridges was told something by the attending ER doctor that would alter the course of her and Porter's lives: "Your son is suffering from a severe reaction to the DPT vaccine that was recently administered, and you need to file a vaccine injury petition with the Vaccine Court."

Sarah did not know what this was all about. As with most parents, little or no information was available in 1994 to inform about those incidents of vaccine injury and what to do in case of any injury. But it did not take long for Dr. Bridges to become aware of the NVICP. She took the doctor's advice, educated herself on her rights as a parent, and contacted a leading vaccine injury attorney in the Minneapolis area, Barbara Ashley, and filed a petition for compensation of injury in the summer of 1994. Porter's injury was brain encephalopathy or brain injury due to the DPT vaccine.

Just a few months after Porter's injury, Dr. Bridges was one of the fortunate parents who filed within the narrow three-year filing period. Most parents are not aware of injuries, much rarer is having another doctor, a pediatrician, or other medical practitioner inform the parent of the vaccine injury program.

But her journey was not an easy one and as she was about to learn, would leave scars on the entire family. The court, after accepting her petition, took nearly five years of back and forth obtaining the necessary medical records, letters, tests, and retests before completing the necessary paperwork to render a decision.

Dr. Bridges felt that the Vaccine Court was requesting retesting in hopes of finding some way to opt out, to find a way to say no, to find some needle in a haystack, to blame some abnormality, in order to state that Porter was not vaccine injured. And she is not alone. Porter's neurologist wrote a letter to the court in support of his vaccine injury. Porter's pediatrician wrote a letter to the court to verify the current condition of Porter, now diagnosed with autism and mental retardation.

Department of Justice attorneys would miss court deadlines and get automatic extensions. In Sarah's mind, why did the DOJ need to drag this out any more?

The Bridges were now saddled with tremendous financial burdens as a result of care for Porter, and were hoping that the Vaccine Court would rule fairly and quickly, just like Congress's intentions. The Bridges were subjected to ridicule by DOJ attorneys, who claimed certain medical documents were ridiculous or crazy. And the court even tried to find a medical test that would show Porter had lycene anemia, an extremely rare condition.

While the court was slowly moving forward, the family structure in the Bridges household was crumbling. Divorce and the constant worrying about the care for Porter took its toll on the family, including Porter's siblings. One of the greatest tragedies that is not reported is the destruction of the family.

But the court took nearly six years to make its ruling. The Bridges were notified in 2000 that Porter was entitled to compensation due to his injuries as a result of his DPT vaccination. It took another year before compensation for pain and suffering, lost income and wages, and unreimbursed medical expenses were funded.

But maybe the toughest part of the entire process with the NVICP was dealing with the life care planner, the court-appointed person who was to determine the future cost of care for Porter. As in most other cases, parents will often criticize with good reason the life care planners as someone who really does not understand the child and the child's specific medical needs. In all fairness, it is tough to determine life-long care for an individual, especially for a vaccine-injured child. There is no magic formula to follow to allocate the necessary funding for the next forty to sixty years. However, when the life care planners do not take the time or effort to get to know the child, to talk with the parents and current medical practitioners who provide care, then these planners are not making decisions in the best interests of the child. In Porter's case, the planner spent one hour with the family to make monetary decisions for the remainder of Porter's life.

Today, the family is on the mend. Nearly twelve years have passed since the court awarded Porter compensation. Porter's brothers and sisters are his biggest supporters. But one has to wonder why families have to be nearly destroyed, why injured victims have be denied essential treatments and therapies, while government attorneys and judges take months and years to determine compensation by arguing over nickels and dimes. The intent of Congress in 1986 was to provide a fair, equitable, and quick resolution to those injured by vaccines. Nothing is fair about the hardship on the family, nothing equitable about trying to find "other" abnormalities to blame other than the vaccine that harmed Porter, and nothing quick about the six years it took to resolve Porter's claim with the NVICP. And as we will find out together, six years is now the new norm replacing the two to three years intended as the new standard for "quick."

Abigail G.

Abigail and her family originally called Arkansas their home. Her mom, Paris, was a nurse for nine years prior to Abigail's birth. All throughout nursing school, all that Paris heard, what she read, and what she was told, was that vaccines are good, they prevent disease, and they protect the young and the frail.

It was an early morning on September 7, 2003, when Abigail was born. It was not your average day and certainly not the average birth of a baby girl. Paris was Group B strep positive and the doctors decided to perform an emergency c-section because Abigail was breech.

Abigail wanted to make an entrance and, boy, did she ever. Paris and her husband welcomed the newest addition to the family. Abigail had a big sister waiting for her. Unlike her younger sister, Natascha did not have any complications at birth nor did she have any reactions to any of the vaccinations that newborns and toddlers receive in the first couple years of their life.

Abigail's parents were college educated, mother was a nurse, and with no complications with her older child's vaccinations, it was decided to proceed with the compulsory vaccinations for newborns.

But this is where the joy and dreams for a new child end and where the ultimate nightmare journey begins for the entire family. Abigail had severe reactions to the vaccinations administered to her at the hospital. Seizures, high fever, and brain inflammation were just a few of the reactions.

Eventually, the doctors placed Abigail in a medically induced coma so they could figure out what went wrong, to plan their next steps, and to hopefully prevent any more pain and suffering to the little girl.

Paris had learned something in nursing school, something that was not complicated at all, and rather simple. But this was what made the difference for Abigail and her future. Paris started a diary from day one. She recorded every event, every detail, every medical treatment administered, and everything that was said.

When Abigail was put into a medically induced coma, Paris set out to start ruling out all possibilities. She was the modern day Sherlock Holmes. Rule out all the impossibilities and what you have left over is the possible. Because of her medical training, she was able to rule out many different possibilities. It became apparent really fast that vaccines were one of the remaining possibilities and causation of her little girl's medical condition. But the doctors were adamantly opposed to this, even stating that there was no possibility.

Now, Paris started to think about the other families that might be going through the same thing as she was. But most of them did not have any medical training, thus they would not have any idea of where to start and what could or could not have caused this.

Paris was determined to find out how the vaccines could cause such an adverse reaction. Her medical training told her that severe reactions were extremely rare, with most reactions being fever and some form of local irritation to the injection site. But she did not recall anyone talking about seizures, high fever for a long period of time, or death. She kept thinking about the doctors: "If you don't admit that it was a possible vaccine injury, how are you going to treat her?"

Paris started her investigation and discovered VAERS. She asked the doctors and the nurses to help her file an adverse reaction with VAERS. They all refused. She did some more research. Using Google, she typed in "vaccine injury" and this led her to the website of NVIC.org (National Vaccine Information Center), a national non-profit established by Barbara Loe Fisher on the top of the search list. The goal of the NVIC was to provide an information and educational resource for vaccine injury, and to provide a contact list of attorneys to help. She learned that she could file an adverse reaction with VAERS herself. But she had never done this before. She kept asking herself, "*How do I do this?*"

She contacted the county health department. She wanted some help to file with VAERS. All she received was some advice to keep her report under 150 words. She felt that they really did not care and were giving her instruction like she was writing an OP/Ed in the local paper.

But because of NVIC.org, she was able to file a report with VAERS and also to contact an experienced attorney who would help her with Abigail's case.

This was the beginning of a long up and down and up journey with the NVICP and the Vaccine Court. Paris had a lot of paperwork, medical documents, and other items to obtain on the behalf of her daughter. This required considerable time.

Over the course of a few years, Abigail's petition made its way through the Vaccine Court. Her attorney, Michael McLaren, was an experienced attorney. Mr. McLaren was an ex-member of the Advisory Commission on Childhood Vaccines (ACCV). The ACCV advises and makes recommendations to the Secretary of Health and Human Services on issues relating to the operation of the National Vaccine Injury Compensation Program (NVICP). So Mr. McLaren has a working knowledge of how the NVICP operates. This is a good advantage for his clients.

During this process, Abigail's parents had to testify to the court, actually to Special Master Richard Abell, about what they believed happened. It was here that the diary surfaced to the surprise of the special master. According to an exchange between the special master and the parents, the diary proved to be one of the deciding factors in awarding damages and ruling in favor of the petitioner, *Abigail G. v. HHS*. It is the family's opinion that Special Master Richard Abell treated them with a great deal of respect and dignity, knowing how difficult the process was for the family.

It took a few years, but Abigail was one of the fortunate few who actually won a compensation award. But the process of moving forward would still be aggravating. As with other cases involving damage awards, it is a painful process to deal with the government's life care planner. The LCP met the family in their home in Rogers, Arkansas, for one day. Just one day to plan for the next sixty to seventy years of Abigail's life. This is one of the biggest complaints of parents toward LCPs. They do not spend enough time with the family to determine a plan for the rest of the child's life. Four or five hours or even a day does not provide enough time to think about the rest of Abigail's future. The parents did not trust the LCP and decided to develop their own plan. They submitted their plan to the court. The respondent, HHS Secretary, through DOJ attorneys, objected to the plan. The process is for both parties to agree upon a plan that will adequately provide for Abigail's medical needs. The government requested a new plan because it was "too beneficial" to the child. Now, one really has to think about what that really means.

Too beneficial? The money is only for the child, not the parents or the rest of the family, so what was the government's real objection, what was their motive for rejecting the plan? It was not their money. They really did not have any skin in the game. This is an area that Congress needs to look into—the actions of the government on how they act regarding life care plans.

But it was not easy for the family either. Their attorney told them that the compensation award was pending and they should not object too much. Sign off on the damage award before it is reduced. Is our federal government threatening families who have won compensation damages in a federal court? It could be.

It was determined that the family was awarded $10,000 in unreimbursed medical expenses for the care of their daughter. The correct amount would be closer to $200,000, all with receipts and supporting documentation. Once again, sign on the dotted line before the award is reduced.

During this negotiated process of settling damages, something became apparent to Paris. And it sickened her tremendously.

During this legal process, kids were not getting the medical help that they truly needed. Parents were losing everything that they owned, selling off valuables to pay medical bills, having cars repossessed, homes foreclosed on, retirement funds liquidated, only to hear, if they are really fortunate, that they have won. Then the reality of finding out that what they won does not even come close to making them whole.

Abigail had medical conditions that made her extremely allergic to most foods and clothing. Her family made a difficult decision to move away from Arkansas and head to California. It was in California that they were able to obtain the food supply that was critical to Abigail's survival. At the time, organic was not available in Arkansas.

The family attorney recommended the trustee to oversee the compensation award for Abigail. Paris became a medical advisor to the trustee to help provide guidance. During this process, Abigail's father was unemployed. The trustee treated the family toughly about their requests for medical treatments for their daughter. Paris felt that the attitude of the trustee toward her husband was not fair and was unwarranted.

There are lot of families who have lost their petition in court, and some who have won. But I have yet to talk to a family that actually won a case and did not suffer long-term financial complications. The damage award in most cases is to reimburse medical expenses, provide for necessary medical treatments, and some pain and suffering. However, that pales in comparison to the financial nightmare that many families face. How do you recover from the home lost in foreclosure due to paying for medical treatments for several years because of a vaccine injury? How do you recover from the mental anguish and pain suffered by the rest of the family? The petitions are taking too long to reach a decision, thus the family and the child suffer. Congress's intent was to provide a quick and fair resolution. I do not see anything quick about a three-to-five-year adjudication of a petition, let alone those that take eight to ten years or longer.

Allison & Chris Chapman

Allison Chapman and her husband, Chris, have three children. CJ, the middle child, was born in December of 1999. A perfectly healthy little boy, CJ regressed into severe autism starting at the age of fifteen months.

At first, Allison did not catch the signs, but soon started to notice. CJ loved a song by Baha Men. He would sing the chorus line, "Who let the dogs out, who, who?" But after receiving his fifteen-month shots, which included the MMR, he was unable to sing along, or even remember the chorus line. This was in March 2001.

Two days after receiving the MMR, CJ was running a constant fever dangerously close to 105°F. Allison cooled him down with tepid water, called the nurse the next morning, and told her that CJ's temperature was down to 103 degrees. The nurse said it was okay. Three days later, CJ developed a full body rash. Allison called the nurse again, discussed it being possible roseola, and decided not to go into the clinic. This is when CJ also developed diarrhea, extreme food intolerances, and the beginning of what was diagnosed a few years later as absence seizures.

After his eighteen-month shots, CJ lost most of his language, he started losing eye contact, and stopped being able to play along with his older sister. The pediatrician mentioned that some kids want to concentrate on gross motor skills as a way to explain CJ's symptoms. CJ was not interested in his favorite song, could not sing it at all. Then the music stopped for all of us. September 11, 2001. Combined with the nervous unknown of what happened with our country and the attack on American soil, Allison was dealing with an unknown medical condition that was attacking CJ.

In October, Allison made an appointment with Early Intervention, who sent out a speech pathologist. Every question she asked had the same answer, "He used to do that but not anymore." The speech pathologist said she believed he had Pervasive Development Disorder. But by two years old, along with another virus, the last of his language left, along with all other previous acquired skills. At this point it was clear that CJ did not have PDD but was in the iron claws of autism.

Allison sought the help of a pediatric neurologist to look into CJ's brain for any clues. An MRI came back clean. The first EEG test results were abnormal. Then a second EEG test came back normal. The neurologist thought autism was a "fad" diagnosis, which is why he did not think CJ had autism. And he completely ignored the first EEG that could have diagnosed his seizures earlier.

With the passage of the new year, Allison started to research not only health care options for her son, but also her options regarding vaccine injury. Previously she had not really paid close attention to the VIS statement provided to a parent for each vaccine that is administered. As Allison and her husband started to look into the option of filing a petition with the National Vaccine Injury Compensation Program, they started to measure the pros and cons that they would face in preparing a petition and seeing it through to the final decision.

With the daunting responsibility of helping CJ recover from the many symptoms of regressive autism, the Chapmans decided to concentrate their efforts, their time, their energy, and their love toward the family. To file a petition with the court to seek compensation for a vaccine injury was not an easy decision to make, one that should not be taken lightly, one that needs to weigh the consequences of dedicating a lot of time and energy away from the family and direct it instead toward the legal system.

The petition process starts with a form that can be filled out by the parents or guardians, plus the need to obtain all medical records, doctors and specialists statements, an attorney, plus the need to keep a constant watch on all court developments, decisions, or motions for additional information.

The Chapmans, like many other families with vaccine-injured children, decided that they needed to concentrate on their child. The demand was so great that they could not bear to fight two wars at the same time. Make no mistake about it, recovering a child from severe regressive autism is like going to war. They just felt that nothing good would come out of the program anyway.

Allison also wanted to be able to tell everyone about their son's journey, the story of recovery from personal perspective. They felt if they had filed a petition with the court, then what they were saying, what they were doing, would be overshadowed by the NVICP and trying to win a decision.

A profound statement by Allison sums up what is happening to many kids who are vaccine injured and regressed into autism. The medical community does not want to listen to the parents. Ask them about their own observations of what is happening to their kids.

The analogy is this: Imagine you and your child are walking down a street and a truck swerves off the road and hits your child. The EMT arrives and asks the parent what happened. But the EMT does not listen to the parent and starts wondering what happened to this boy. The answer is right there in front of you. Ask the parent what happened. What have you noticed about your child? No one believes the parent.

Caitlyn Hoiberg: Her Sister's Cheerleader

Caitlyn was born into a medically savvy household. Her mother, Sarah, always researched every medical technique, vaccine, and procedure that was being administered to a member of the family. Caitlyn's maternal grandmother was holistic.

When Sarah brought Caitlyn or her older sister, Laura, to the pediatric office for well-baby visits and vaccinations, Sarah always asked for the Vaccine Information Statement, or VIS. The pediatrician, with a wonderful bedside manner, gave Sarah time to read the VIS and was always available to answer any questions. There was no rushing to administer the recommended vaccinations. The doctor would wait until Sarah and her daughters were ready.

Caitlyn's pediatrician assured her mother and older sister that in his thirty-five-plus years of practice, he had never seen or witnessed any problems such as seizures or anaphylactic shock. Sarah trusted her pediatrician completely. Because of Sarah's constant research, she knew the concerning vaccine was the MMR. But on this day, little Caitlyn was to receive the DTaP vaccine. There was little about it in the news, so she did not question the side effects of this vaccine.

And this is the day that would define the Hoibergs, that would measure their resiliency. This is the day, like for so many other families, where the world is turned upside down on you.

The very next day, Sarah found Caitlyn laying on her bed, eyes wide open, her left side of her body stiff as a board, yet her right side limp. She was having seizures. Frantically, Sarah called 911 and told the dispatcher that her little girl was having seizures.

As the paramedics arrived, Sarah demanded to ride with her little girl to the hospital. In the ambulance, she told one of the paramedics that Caitlyn just received her shots the day before. And Sarah could sense that the paramedic really did not believe her, that the vaccines would not cause this. Even the next question to Sarah seemed odd. The paramedic asked if the seizures were a normal routine for Caitlyn. As if the paramedic did not hear what Sarah said.

In the ER, Caitlyn began to have more seizures and the doctors could not stop them. So little Caitlyn was admitted to the hospital. The doctors did not believe that the vaccines would cause seizures. They began to treat her and perform many, many tests for every known infectious disease and medical condition, and even performed a spinal tap.

The admitting doctor told Sarah and her husband Chris to call all family members to come up and say goodbye to Caitlyn. The message was "there was nothing that they could do to stop the seizures." Caitlyn was then placed into a medically induced coma for five days.

When she came out of the coma, she started to have seizures. The doctors were puzzled, mentioning that something was wrong with her brain but they did not know what it was and how to correct it.

It was a couple of days later, now day seven in the hospital, that a neurologist approached Sarah and suggested that Caitlyn could have been vaccine injured and told her how to file a VAERS report. Caitlyn's grandmother, being from a holistic background, reached out to an old friend who knew about vaccine injuries and the necessary procedures to file a petition.

Through an aggressive search, they found a local law firm in Florida and an attorney, Alan Pickert. Mr. Pickert was interested in representing Caitlyn, but instructed Sarah that they had to wait six months. Since one of the conditions to file a petition is that the injury must last for a minimum of six months.

During the interim, Mr. Pickert started building a case, obtaining the necessary medical records. He was not wasting time and had the petition ready to go once the six-month period had expired.

The petition of *Caitlyn Hoiberg v. HHS* was filed March 10, 2006. And the petition was awarded compensation September 24, 2007. This is unusual since most cases, especially those dealing with complex medical conditions, seizure disorders, obtaining medical records, medical expert testimony, take three to four years or even longer. This case was adjudicated in eighteen months, mainly because of the aggressive attorney, Alan Pickert, who worked feverishly gathering all the necessary documents while waiting for the six-month period to expire.

Caitlyn's attorney would constantly update the family on the status of the petition to provide some insight and hope during the process. Within three months of filing, Pickert called Sarah and told her that the respondent (HHS) would concede the case. And the difficult work of finding an appropriate life care planner began.

In May 2007, both the respondent's pair of life care planners, along with Terry, representing Caitlyn, arrived at the Hoiberg residence to interview the family and to properly assess the current and future needs of Caitlyn.

The interview process was difficult on the family, as it is a very exhaustive and probing process. In order to ascertain a reasonable "lost earnings" estimate, the parents are interviewed to determine their own potential lifetime earnings including educational background, current careers, and financial status.

A reasonable question can be asked: Can a child surpass the accomplishments of their parents? What can be said of a child who becomes a doctor from a family that lives in poverty? How about a child who does not rise above the parents' education and career achievements? It is a tricky process to determine lost wages. The LCP also assumes that any current health insurance maintained by the family must continue.

During the LCP interview, the respondent's representative was engaging and suggested a generous treatment and therapy financial plan. But that caught the attention of Mr. Pickert. And it should have. When the respondent's LCP was submitted, it appeared that the entire plan was reversed by pressure to reduce the financial care. It was like DOJ did not care what was in the best interests of the injured child. And this is the case for so many petitioners: the headaches, the anguish of having to deal with a plan that is not sufficient to provide the necessary medical care for the injured child.

During a conference call with both parties, Mr. Pickert mentioned that the LCP submitted by the respondent was not worth the paper it was printed on. And the court agreed with Sarah, as the special master, George Hastings, instructed the parties to work out the differences.

During this entire process, an outside observer would have to wonder why the LCP process was so adversarial. It is difficult to plan for the financial needs of a vaccine-injured child. One of the biggest points of friction generally occurs when LCPs have to interview the family to determine future costs for ongoing medical care.

Fortunately, Mr. Pickert had his own LCP submit a plan to the court that countered the government's plan. A lot of times, the petitioner, even armed with their own plan, would have to accept the life care plan submitted by the government. But not this time, and fortunately for Caitlyn, the plan would provide the necessary medical treatment for the rest of her life.

September of 2007 rolled around and the Hoibergs were at their breaking point. Dealing with the day-to-day medical and therapeutic needs of their daughter and not knowing whether the court was going to resolve the issue of a life care plan was taking its toll.

The Hoibergs were called into their attorney's office to review paperwork. The mood was solemn. Chris and Sarah were expecting the worst, that the parties could not reach an agreement. Mr. Pickert approached them with settlement papers and a big smile.

Sarah finally was able to relax, to think about Caitlyn finally being financially taken care of for the rest of her life. But there was more work to be done: set up guardianship accounts, and obtain state certification of guardianship.

Funding was completed a month later. The normal time is six months or greater depending on the establishment of trust accounts or issues with guardianships. The entire process, from the moment of meeting Alan Pickert for the first time, to the filing process, to the settlement, was done over a period of eighteen months, as if there was some divine intervention for this little girl. Eighteen months is a short period of time. Similar cases can take as much as four to ten years to settle. There are many cases where the LCP process alone takes a couple of years.

The terms of the settlement were good for Caitlyn, a large amount in the form of an annuity, plus sufficient money for pain and suffering plus lost earnings. But that money is for Caitlyn and not for use by the rest of the family. Sarah would have to keep reminding her friends and family members that they do not have the money to go on extended or elaborate vacations. The court settlement was for Caitlyn.

Now my question to Sarah is, and it is the same that I have asked several other parents: What would it be like if you did not have the financial resources such as good health insurance to provide care for Caitlyn until the court decided in favor of your little girl? Would Caitlyn have suffered? Sarah quickly answered that she does not want to think about that scenario, but it is a common thought.

For many of the injured children of parents who do not have the financial resources to provide medical care during the petition process that could take three, four, or even eight years or more before a decision is made, what happens to the child? The court and HHS need to recognize this issue and start to address it. There is no need for the child to suffer while the court is adjudicating the petition.

Sarah and Chris, like many other parents, had high hopes and big dreams for their children. And those dreams were quickly erased in 2006 when Caitlyn received her DTaP vaccine.

Her big sister Laura has become her guardian, a caretaker, a role that she shouldn't have had to assume, but has accepted. There have been so many times that Laura has come to the rescue of her mother, when Sarah was having a bad day, by quietly telling her, that is okay mommy, I will take care of Caitlyn. Little do we know what we can expect from a brother or sister, who might step up and become that guardian, that caretaker. That should not be their role, not yet, but it is one they often gladly accept. Laura is a godsend, an angel for Caitlyn.

Laura not only has to watch over her little sister, but she is also trying to become a competitive ice skater. In a world where just the wrong angle of the blade touching the ice could throw the balance of the skater to the ice, what is more important to Laura is to have Caitlyn sitting in the stands, cheering her on, being the cheerleader for her older sister, her guardian angel.

Sarah believes in her heart that God has big and wonderful plans for Caitlyn.

ACKNOWLEDGMENTS

I have many people to thank and recognize for helping me and encouraging my work. Over the past few years, I have spent a tremendous amount of time researching case decisions and court dockets, reading many published articles, and discussing policy with elected officials.

For the last three years, I have talked with many families who have experienced the petition process of the program, listening to their private journey, discussing their opinions and comments, reliving the ordeals of many who have lost family members, and witnessing the inner strength and will to go on for those families that have suffered a great tragedy. To all of you, the families that have opened up their lives, their hearts, and innermost feelings, I want to thank you and wish only the best for you and your family.

To my wife, Robyne, thank you for giving me the time and latitude to proceed with this project. To my son, Austin, every day you ask me how the book is coming along, when will it be published, and every night before you go to bed, you ask me to get some sleep and not to stay up too late; I want to thank you so very much and for helping take care of your brother. To my son, Nicholas, my inspiration for my autism advocacy, I pray that someday we can sit down on a park bench and you can ask me about this book. To my family, all my love.

A special thank you to Lou Conte and our daily phone calls; to Mary Holland, thank you for your guidance and wisdom; to John

Stone and our across-the-Big Pond discussions; and to several attorneys who practice in the NVICP, including Robert Krakow, John McHugh, Renee Gentry, Robert Homer, Andrew Downing, Ed Krause, William Dobreff, Barbara Ashley, Sherry Drew, and Anne Toale.

NOTES

How Did We Get Here?

1. http://supreme.justia.com/cases/federal/us/197/11/
2. http://constitution.laws.com/preamble/jacobson-v-massachu-setts-1905#sthash.J4pc736F.dpuf
3. http://www.sfgate.com/health/article/When-polio-vaccine-backfired-Tainted-batches-2677525.php
4. Ibid.
5. Ibid.
6. *Gottsdanker v. Cutter Laboratories*, 182 Cal.App.2d 602, 6 Cal.Rptr. 320, 79 A.L.R.2d 290 (Cal.App. 1 Dist. Jul 12, 1960)
7. Ibid.
8. "The Plague of Causation in the National Childhood Vaccine Injury Act"—Betsy Grey
9. *Davis v. Wyeth Laboratories, Inc.*, 399 F.2d 121 (9th Cir.(Idaho) Jan 22, 1968)
10. http://biotech.law.lsu.edu/cases/vaccines/davis_v_wyeth_labo-ratories_brief.htm
11. Ibid.
12. http://biotech.law.lsu.edu/cases/vaccines/reyes_v_wyeth_labo-ratories.htm
13. "The Plague of Causation in the National Childhood Vaccine Injury Act"—Betsy Grey
14. http://biotech.law.lsu.edu/cases/vaccines/reyes_v_wyeth_labo-ratories_brief.htm

15. "The Plague of Causation in the National Childhood Vaccine Injury Act"—Betsy Grey

16. Ibid.

17. "The Plague of Causation in the National Childhood Vaccine Injury Act"—Betsy Grey

18. *Alvarez v. US*, 495 F. Supp. 1188, 1190 (D. Colo. 1980)

19. "The 800 Pound Gorilla Sleeps: The Federal Government's Lackadaisical Liability and Compensation Policies in the Context of Pre-Event Vaccine Immunization Programs," Michael Greenberger, citing National Swine Flu Immunization Program of 1976.

20. Ibid.

21. *Wallace v. United States*, 669 F. 2d 947

22. Ibid.

23. http://blogs.discovermagazine.com/bodyhorrors/2013/09/30/public-health-legacy-1976-swine-flu/

24. http://articles.latimes.com/2009/apr/27/science/sci-swine-history27

25. Ibid.

26. Ibid.

27. "The Plague of Causation in the National Childhood Vaccine Injury Act"—Betsy Grey

28. *60 Minutes* story, https://www.youtube.com/watch?v=8elE7Ct1jWw

29. Ibid.

30. Ibid.

31. Ibid.

32. "The Epidemic that Never Was"—Richard Neustadt and Harvey Fineberg

33. Ibid.

34. Ibid.

35. Dept. of HEW press release—December 16, 1976

36. *60 Minutes* story, https://www.youtube.com/watch?v=8elE7Ct1jWw

37. Ibid.
38. Swine Flu Immunization Products Liability Litigation, 446 F. Supp. 244 (Jud.Pan.Mult.Lit.1978)
39. *60 Minutes* interview, aired Nov. 1979
40. "Vaccine: The Controversial Story of the Medicine's Greatest Lifesaver"—Arthur Allen
41. Ibid.
42. Ibid.
43. http://www.historyofvaccines.org/content/articles/vaccine-injury-compensation-programs
44. Ibid.
45. Ibid.
46. US Department of Health and Human Services
47. "Vaccine: The Controversial Story of the Medicine's Greatest Lifesaver"—Arthur Allen
48. Ibid.
49. *The Oxford Handbook of the Economics of the Biopharmaceutical Industry*
50. Ibid.
51. Ibid.
52. "Vaccine: The Controversial Story of the Medicine's Greatest Lifesaver"—Arthur Allen
53. "The Plague of Causation in the National Childhood Vaccine Injury Act"—Betsy Grey

Congress and the National Vaccine Injury Compensation Program

1. S.R. 2117, 98th Congress (1983)
2. H.R. 5810, 98th Congress (1984)
3. Ibid.
4. H.R. 5810, 98th Congress (1984)
5. "The Plague of Causation in the National Childhood Vaccine Injury Act"—Betsy Grey

6. Ibid.
7. H.R. 1780, 99th Congress (1985)
8. H.R. 1780, 99th Congress (1985)
9. "The Plague of Causation in the National Childhood Vaccine Injury Act"—Betsy Grey
10. Ibid.
11. National Vaccine Injury Compensation Program, http://www.hhs.gov/asl/testify/t990928b.html
12. Ibid.
13. Ibid.
14. S. 1744, 99th Congress (1986)
15. *New York Times*, "Reagan signs bill on Drug Exports and Payment for Vaccine Injuries," Robert Pear, Nov. 15, 1986
16. Ibid.
17. Ibid.
18. S. 1744, 99th Congress (1986)
19. "The Plague of Causation in the National Childhood Vaccine Injury Act"—Betsy Grey
20. S. 1744, 99th Congress (1986)
21. "The Plague of Causation in the National Childhood Vaccine Injury Act"—Betsy Grey
22. Barbara Loe Fisher—testimony to US House Government Reform Cmte—August 3, 1999
23. S. 1744, 99th Congress (1986)

Congressional Oversight

1. GAO Report to Congress, March 2000—Vaccine Injury Trust Fund
2. GAO Report to Congress, Dec. 1999—Vaccine Injury Compensation
3. Ibid.
4. Barbara Loe Fisher testimony to House subcommittee, Sept. 28, 1999

5. GAO Report to Congress, Dec. 1999—Vaccine Injury Compensation

6. "Fixing the Flaws in the Federal Vaccine Injury Compensation Program," Peter Meyers, 2011

7. GAO Report to Congress, Dec. 1999—Vaccine Injury Compensation

8. Court Appointed Experts—Digital Access to Scholarship at http://dash.harvard.edu/bitstream/handle/1/10018993/pan-g03REDACTED.html?sequence=2

9. House Report 106-977—HRPT106-977—GPO, http://www.gpo.gov/fdsys/pkg/CRPT-106hrpt977/html/CRPT-106hrpt977.htm

10. GAO Report to Congress, Dec. 1999—Vaccine Injury Compensation

11. House Report 106-977—HRPT106-977—GPO, http://www.gpo.gov/fdsys/pkg/CRPT-106hrpt977/html/CRPT-106hrpt977.htm

12. GAO Report to Congress, Dec. 1999—Vaccine Injury Compensation

13. Guillain-Barré Syndrome is an acute polyneuropathy, a disorder affecting the peripheral nervous system. Ascending paralysis, weakness beginning in the feet and hands and migrating toward the trunk, is the most typical symptom, and some subtypes cause changes in sensation or pain, as well as dysfunction of the autonomic nervous system. It can cause life-threatening complications, in particular if the respiratory muscles are affected or if the autonomic nervous system is involved. The disease is usually triggered by an infection.

14. HHS Inspector General Report, December 1992

15. HHS Inspector General Report, December 1992

16. IRS Code, Section 9602 (b)

17. Vaccine Injury Compensation: Program Challenged to Settle, http://www.gpo.gov/fdsys/pkg/GAOREPORTS-HEHS-00-8/html/GAOREPORTS-HEHS-00- 8.htm

18. http://www.treasurydirect.gov/govt/reports/tfmp/vaccomp/vac-comp.htm

19. US GAO—"Vaccine Injury Trust Fund: Revenue Exceeds Current Needs for Paying Claims"; http://www.gao.gov/products/HEHS-00-67

20. Ibid.

21. Ibid.

22. US GAO—"Vaccine Injury Trust Fund: Revenue Exceeds Current Needs for Paying Claims"; http://www.gao.gov/products/HEHS-00-67

23. Ibid.

24. GAO Report to Congress, Dec. 1999—Vaccine Injury Compensation

De Minimis

1. 42 US Code §300aa–11—Petitions for compensation http://www.law.cornell.edu/uscode/text/42/300aa-11

2. Ibid.

3. Ibid.

4. Ibid.

5. Federal Register: National Vaccine Injury Compensation, https://www.federalregister.gov/articles/2001/07/13/01-16814/national-vaccine-injury-compensation-program-revisions-and-additions-to-the-vaccine-injury-table

6. "Article: Native Americans and the Vaccine Act: Excluding Those We Found Here," https://litigation-essentials.lexisnexis.com/webcd/app?action=DocumentDisplay&crawlid=1&doctype=cite&docid=46+Am.+U.L.+Rev.+1935&srctype=smi&srcid=3B15&key=e6dedbcb483dab86f74ca83cd73de0ea

7. Ibid.

8. Ibid.

9. www.wcl.american.edu/journal/lawrev/46/leachtxt.html

10. Victor E. Schwartz, Mark A. Behrens and Leavy Mathews III, "Federalism and Federal Liability Reform: The United States

Constitution Supports Reform," 36 Harv. J. on Legis. 269, 297 (1997), citing *Black v. Sec'y HHS*

11. *La Londe v. Secretary of HHS*

Pro Se

1. http://www.jud6.org/generalpublic/RepresentingYourself/CourtInfoAndResource/Prosedef.htm
2. *Haines v. Kerner*, 404 US 519, 520-21 (1972)
3. No-Fault Vaccine Insurance: Lessons from the National Vaccine Injury Compensation Program

Statute of Limitations

1. Section 300aa-16(a)(2) of the Vaccine Act
2. Section 300aa-16(b) of the Vaccine Act
3. http://www.hrsa.gov/vaccinecompensation/vaccinetable.html
4. Ibid.
5. http://www.ebcala.org/areas-of-law/vaccine-law/case-comment-on-cloer-v-hhs, Kim Mac Rosenberg
6. http://definitions.uslegal.com/e/equitable-tolling/
7. Ibid.
8. *Herbert v. HHS*
9. *Brice v. HHS*, 240 F. 3rd 1367, 1370 (Fed Cir. 2001)
10. 42 C.F.R. 100.3(a)
11. 42 U.S.C. 300aa-16(a)(2)
12. Section 300aa-11(c) of the Vaccine Act
13. Interviews conducted with parents in person and by telephone
14. *Estepp v HHS*
15. Ibid.
16. Mark Rogers, Civil Torts Division of DOJ, presentation to the ACCV meeting March 2007
17. Ibid.

18. *Markovich v. HHS*
19. Ibid.
20. Ibid.
21. *Goetz v. HHS*
22. *Setnes v. HHS*
23. Leonard Pertnoy, "A Child's View of Recovery Under The National Childhood Vaccine Act, or 'He Who Hesitates is Lost,'" *Montana Law Review* 59(1998), citing *Pertnoy v. HHS*, # 95-218v, Special Master Laura Millman
24. Ibid.
25. The National Vaccine Injury Compensation Program, A Program Evaluation. Betty Pang (2003)
26. "Strong Medicine: Procedural Limitations and Their Effect on Vaccine Injury Claims," Justin Roller
27. *Staley v. HHS*
28. *Order of Railroad Telegraphers v. Railway Express Agency*, 321 US 342, 349, 64 St. Ct. 582, 586, L.Ed 788

Redaction Rule 18(b)

1. *Langland v. HHS*, Federal Court of Claims, Special Master Lord order, February 3, 2011
2. Vaccine Act of 1986, adopted rules of procedure
3. *Langland v. HHS*, Federal Court of Claims, Special Master Lord order, February 3, 2011
4. Ibid.
5. Ibid.
6. Ibid.
7. Ibid.
8. Ibid.
9. Section 2112(b)(2) of the PHS Act, 42 U.S.C. 300aa-12(b)(2), requires the Sec'y of HHS, within 30 days after receiving service of any petition filed under sections 2111, to publish notice of such petition in the Federal Register

10. *Langland v. HHS*, Federal Court of Claims, Special Master Lord order, February 3, 2011
11. Ibid.
12. *C.S. v. HHS*, Court of Federal Claims 07-293v, Special Master Daria Zane decision August 19, 2013
13. Ibid.
14. *A.K. v. HHS*, Court of Federal Claims 09-605v, Special Master Dorsey decision January 17, 2013
15. Ibid.
16. *Mary Browning v. HHS*, Federal Court of Claims 02-928v, 02-929v, 07-453v Special Master Lord October 5, 2010

Proving Off-Table Injuries

1. "Fixing the Vaccine Act's Structural Moral Hazard" – Brandon Boxler, *Pepperdine Dispute Resolution Law Journal*
2. *Lowry ex rel. Lowry v. Sec'y of HHS*
3. The Plague of Causation in the NCVIA
4. In the US legal system, "arbitrary and capricious" is one of the basic standards for review of appeals. Under the "arbitrary and capricious" standard, the finding of a lower court will not be disturbed unless it has no reasonable basis. When a judge makes a decision without reasonable grounds or adequate consideration of the circumstances, it is said to be arbitrary and capricious and can be invalidated by an appellate court on that ground. In other words, there should be an absence of a rational connection between the facts found and the choice made. There should be a clear error of judgment, an action not based upon consideration of relevant factors and so is arbitrary, capricious, an abuse of discretion, or otherwise not in accordance with law or taken without observance of procedure required by law. US Legal Definition. http://definitions.uslegal.com/a/arbitrary-and-capricious/

5. The Plague of Causation in the NCVIA
6. *Grant v. HHS*
7. The Plague of Causation in the NCVIA
8. Ibid.
9. Ibid.
10. *Jay v. HHS*
11. *Golub v. HHS*
12. The Plague of Causation in the NCVIA
13. Ibid.
14. Ibid.
15. Ibid.
16. Ibid.
17. Ibid.
18. *Shyface v. HHS*
19. *Grant v. HHS*
20. Ibid.
21. *Shyface v. HHS*
22. *Althen v. HHS*, CAFC decision
23. *Grant v. HHS*, 956 F.2d 1144, 1148 (Fed. Cir. 1992)
24. 42 U.S.C. 300aa-3333(4)
25. H.R. Rep. No. 99-908, at 1 (2d Session 1986), reprinted in 1986 U.S.C.C.A.N. 6344, 6356)
26. 42 U.S.C. 300aa11(c)(1)(c)(i)-(ii)
27. *Misasi v. HHS*
28. *Whitecotton v. HHS*, CAFC remand decision
29. 42 U.S.C. 300aa13(a)(1)
30. *Whitecotton v. HHS*
31. *Althen v. HHS*, 418 F.3d at 1278

Death

1. 42 U.S.C. § 300aa-15(a)(2)
2. *Zatuchni v. HHS*
3. *Graves v. HHS*

4. Ibid.

5. Ibid.

6. *Graves v. HHS*

7. Ibid.

8. Ibid,

9. Ibid.

10. US Court of Federal Claims, *Graves v. HHS* 02-1211v, Judge Merow opinion and order July 5, 2011

11. US Court of Federal Claims, *Graves v. HHS* 02-1211v, SM Moran decision on remand, August 3, 2012

12. *Zatuchni v. Sec'y of HHS*, 516 F. 3d 1312, 1318 (Fed. Cir. 2008)

13. 2012 WL 1611578

14. US Court of Federal Claims, *Graves v. HHS* 02-1211v, Senior Judge Merow Opinion of Feb. 25, 2013

15. Ibid.

16. US Court of Federal Claims, *Graves v. HHS* 02-1211v, Senior Judge Merow Opinion of Feb. 25, 2013

17. Ibid.

18. Ibid.

19. Ibid.

20. *Clifford v. HHS*

21. Ibid.

22. Ibid.

23. Ibid.

Yates Hazlehurst, Michelle Cedillo, and the OAP

1. SM Gary Golkiewicz General Order #1, Autism Master File

2. Ibid.

3. *Leroy v. HHS*, SM Golkiewicz (2002)

4. Chief Special Master Gary Golkiewicz issued the Autism General Order #1, to address a method for handling the large and growing number of petitions filed in the NVICP.

5. Autism Master File—Ruling concerning Petitioners' Second Motion to Compel

6. Ibid.

7. Ibid.

8. Vaccine Act—300aa-12(d)(3)(B)

9. Ibid.

10. Appendix B of the Rules of the Court of Federal Claims

11. www.cdc.gov/vaccinesafety/activities/vsd.html

12. Autism Update—May 25, 2007, placed in the Autism Master File, Court of Federal Claims.

13. Autism Master File—Ruling concerning Petitioners' Second Motion to Compel

14. This phrase is often found in legal pleadings and writings to specify one example out of many possibilities.

15. Autism Master File—Ruling concerning Petitioners' Second Motion to Compel

16. Ibid.

17. Ibid.

18. Ibid.

19. Autism Update—May 25, 2007, placed in the Autism Master File, Court of Federal Claims.

20. Ibid.

21. Ibid.

22. Ibid.

23. *Cedillo v. HHS*, Exhibit FF

24. Dr. Zimmerman's letter of April 24, 2007, sent to DOJ re: Cedillo case

25. Interview with Rolf Hazlehurst

26. Autism Update—May 25, 2007, placed in the Autism Master File, Court of Federal Claims.

27. *Hazlehurst v. HHS*, transcript of oral arguments, Oct. 18, 2007

28. *Poling v. HHS*, Rule 4-C report, filed November 9, 2007
29. Ibid.
30. Interview with Rolf Hazlehurst
31. Ibid.
32. Ibid.
33. Ibid.
34. Ibid.
35. Interview with Rolf Hazlehurst and examining Yates's medical records, which were introduced as evidence in the Hazlehurst hearing.
36. *Mead v. HHS*, SM Campbell-Smith decision, May 2010
37. Ibid.
38. *Poling v. HHS*, Order deferring ruling on Petitioner's motion for complete transparency of proceedings.
39. Ibid.
40. *Cedillo v. HHS*, Special Master George Hastings decision
41. Definition: Latin term meaning "friend of the court." The name for a brief filed with the court by someone who is not a party to the case.
42. *Cedillo v. HHS*, US Court of Appeals for the Federal Circuit, Brief of Amici Curiae, Mary Holland, Esq., EBCALA, in support of Cedillo, Jan. 25, 2010
43. US MMR Litigation—The Truth—And was Dr. Stephen Bustin a reliable witness?
44. Vaccine Epidemic
45. Brian Deer's presentation to University of Wisconsin–LaCrosse
46. Brian Deer's presentation to University of Wisconsin–LaCrosse
47. *Hazlehurst v. HHS*, Federal Circuit Court of Appeals, oral arguments
48. Rolf Hazlehurst's written testimony to Congress, Oversight and Government Reform, submitted 2013

Is It Genetic or Is It Vaccination?

1. *Forbes*, Alice Walton, "Parental Age, Especially the Father's, Is Linked to Genetic Mutation in the Child." http://www.forbes.com/sites/alicegwalton/2012/08/24/parental-age-especially-the-fathers-is-linked-to-genetic-mutations-in-the-child/

2. Funded by Bionomics, a research and development company for new treatments of cancer and serious disorders of the central nervous system. "Unanswered Questions," Holland, Krakow, Conte, Colin (2011)

3. S. F. Berkovic et al., "De-Novo Mutations of the Sodium Channel Gene SCN1A in Alleged Vaccine Encephalopathy: A Retrospective Study," *Lancet Neurology* Lancet Neurol. 2006 June; 5(6):488-92

4. "Unanswered Questions," Holland, Krakow, Conte, Colin (2011)

5. "Effects of vaccination on onset and outcome of Dravet syndrome: a retrospective study," Anne McIntosh, PhD, *The Lancet Neurology*, 2010. http://www.thelancet.com/pdfs/journals/laneur/PIIS1474442210701071.pdf

6. "Effects of vaccination on onset and outcome of Dravet syndrome: a retrospective study," Anne McIntosh, PhD, *The Lancet Neurology*, 2010. http://www.thelancet.com/pdfs/journals/laneur/PIIS1474442210701071.pdf

7. Age of Autism, "Vaccine May Trigger Early Start of Infant Epilepsy, Vaccine Apologist Shrugs Off Science," May 6, 2010, Maggie Fox and Krittivas Mukherjee. http://www.ageofautism.com/2010/05/vaccine-may-trigger-early-start-of-infant-epilepsy-vaccine-apologist-shrugs-off-science.html

8. Yuval Shafrir, "Vaccination and Dravet Syndrome," 9 *Lancet Neurology* 1147-48 (2010), available at http://www.thelancet.com/journals/laneur/article/PIIS1474-4422(10)70288-X/fulltext

9. Federal Court of Claims, *Hammitt v. HHS*, Judge Wheeler order and opinion

10. The Vaccine Act requires the respondent to file a Rule 4(c) report with the special master summarizing the evidence presented and addressing any legal issues the case presents. The Division of Vaccine Injury Compensation (DVIC), an agency within HRSA, reviews each petition that is filed with the program and coordinates with the DOJ attorney assigned to the case. These reports are confidential and are not made public.

11. Federal Court of Claims, *Hammitt v. HHS*, Judge Wheeler order and opinion

12. *Snyder v. HHS*, May 27, 2011

13. *Snyder v. HHS*, Braden Opinion, November 2011

14. *Deribeaux v. HHS*, Millman decision Dec 17, 2007

15. Kawasaki disease is "a syndrome of unknown etiology, usually affecting infants and young children, associated with vasculitis of the large coronary vessels and numerous other systemic signs, including fever, conjunctival infection, changes of the oropharyngeal mucosa, cervical lymphadenopathy, and maculoerythematous skin eruption that becomes confluent and bright red in a glove-and-sock distribution; the skin becomes indurated and edematous and often desquamates from the fingers and toes." *Dorland's Illustrated Medical Dictionary*, 30th ed. (2003), p.536.

16. *The West Australian*, "Old Vaccine for Whooping Cough, 'is best,'" Cathy O'Leary, Medical Editor, March 26, 2014

17. *Scientific American*, "Shooting the Wheeze: Whooping Cough Vaccine Falls Short of Previous Shot's Protection," Tara Haelle, May 21, 2013.

Moving Too Fast?

1. Off-the-record interviews with attorneys who are members of the Vaccine Bar.

2. Off-the-record interview with attorney who represents several petitioners claiming Gardasil caused vaccine-related injury.

3. http://www.uscfc.uscourts.gov/

4. http://www.uscfc.uscourts.gov/

5. http://www.hrsa.gov/vaccinecompensation/vaccinetable.html

6. US Federal Circuit Court of Appeals, *Althen v. Secretary of HHS*, 04-5146 (U.S.Ct.App, Fed. Cir. 2005)

7. Ibid.

8. *Capizzano v. HHS*, 2006

9. *Flores v. HHS,* 2013

10. Ibid.

11. Ibid.

12. Ibid.

13. Ibid.

14. *Flores v. HHS*—Special Master George Hastings

15. "Postlicensure Safety Surveillance for HPV Vaccine," published by JAMA, August 19, 2009, Vol. 302, No. 7. Lists pulmonary embolism as a serious reaction. Mayo Clinic defines pulmonary embolism as "Pulmonary Embolism is when one or more pulmonary arteries in your lungs become blocked. In most cases, pulmonary embolism is caused by blood clots."

16. *Incze v. HHS*, 2012

17. *Incze v. HHS*, 2012

18. *Collins v. HHS*, 2013

Dare to Reform

1. 42 U.S.C. 300aa-16(a)

2. 42 U.S.C. 300aa-16(a)(3)

3. Peter Meyers, "Fixing the Flaws in the NVICP," *Administrative Law Review*, Fall 2011

4. Cliff Shoemaker, testimony to House Government Reform Committee, 1999

5. Peter Meyers, "Fixing the Flaws in the NVICP," *Administrative Law Review*, Fall 2011

6. Ibid.

7. Ibid.

8. *Stevens v. HHS*

9. 42 U.S.C. 300aa-16(a)(3)

10. http://www.hrsa.gov/vaccinecompensation/processincrease.pdf

11. "Sept. 11 Victim Compensation Fund, Take Two: New Rules for First Responders Web. April 2, 2014 http://www.cpradr. org/Resources/ALLCPRArticles/tabid/265/ID/719/Sept-11-Victim-Compensation-Fund-Take-Two-New-Rules-for-First-Responders-June-24.aspx

12. Kenneth Feinberg speech, Negotiating the September 11 Victim Compensation Fund

13. Ibid.

14. Ibid.

15. *Langland v. HHS*, Lord decision Feb. 3, 2011

16. RCFC 5.2(a) permits redaction of certain identifying information, specifically, the name of a minor child, which may be redacted to initials, and an individual's birth date. See E-Government Act of 2002, Pub. L. No. 107-347, § 205(a)-(c), 116 Stat. 2899, 2913 (codified as amended at 44 U.S.C. § 3501 note (2006)); RCFC 5.2(a). No further redaction of identifying information is required by the E-Government Act or the rules implementing it.

17. http://www.hrsa.gov/vaccinecompensation/statisticsreports. html#Note:2

18. *Langland v. HHS*, Lord decision Feb. 3, 2011

19. In the United States Court of Federal Claims. (n.d.). Retrieved from http://www.mctlawyers.com/vaccine-cases/vaccine-case-results/10-802V-flu-shot-frozen-shoulder-syndrome.pdf

20. RCFC 12(b)(1). Petition bears the burden of establishing subject matter jurisdiction.

21. ACCV meeting, Workgroup report of March 2007. ACCV voted 8-1 in favor of this recommendation.

Index